HIV/AIDS in Rural Communities

Fayth M. Parks · Gregory S. Felzien
Sally Jue

Editors

HIV/AIDS in Rural Communities

Research, Education, and Advocacy

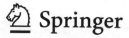 Springer

Editors
Fayth M. Parks
Department of Leadership, Technology,
  and Human Development
Georgia Southern University
Statesboro, GA
USA

Gregory S. Felzien
Division of Health Protection/IDI-HIV
Georgia Department of Public Health
Atlanta, GA
USA

Sally Jue
Organizational and Diversity Consultant
Los Angeles, CA
USA

ISBN 978-3-319-85862-3   ISBN 978-3-319-56239-1   (eBook)
DOI 10.1007/978-3-319-56239-1

Printed on acid-free paper

This Springer imprint is published by Springer Nature
The registered company is Springer International Publishing AG
The registered company address is: Gewerbestrasse 11, 6330 Cham, Switzerland

Foreword

The editors, Parks, Felzien, and Jue, have produced and put forward a critically informative book on HIV and rural health. Through their lens and along with their expert co-authors, they have provided a treatise on understanding and addressing one of the major challenges of HIV and public health in America today—the nuanced and transecting reality of rural health dynamics. In an effective manner, they present not only the current status of HIV in rural America, but also the key challenges, tested solutions, and the research that is needed as a means to hit this public health crisis head on now and for effective planning, focus, resource allocation, and program and services implementation going forward.

If we are to meet the UNAIDS 90-90-90 goals and the indices set out by the National HIV/AIDS Strategy, we must understand and garner our efforts in fighting HIV and AIDS in rural communities. And what this really means is if we are to successfully reach those at risk and those in need who are often left behind, or simply left out, due to geographic layout and related factors, we must understand and focus on research, programs, services, and policies toward addressing the challenges of rural HIV risks and transmission alongside AIDS treatment and care.

The nature and impact of a changing economy often working against rural towns and communities; forms of social isolation, stigma and other mental health challenges; the crisis of opioid, alcohol and other substance use in rural settings; the lack of training, education, and health resources along with an all too often scarcity of HIV specialists are impacting HIV in rural America. But, as brought forth in this book, there is also a rising awareness and level of understanding that is taking hold. This includes the recognition and use of proven HIV prevention techniques such as syringe exchange programs and tailored education as well as new innovative approaches, including telehealth and HIV specific prevention and treatment apps that are now available and being utilized. The need for seek, test, treat, and retain is as relevant for HIV/AIDS in rural communities as anywhere; and, addressing the gaps in the HIV/AIDS treatment cascade is as critical in the rural parts as in the rest of America. Treatment as prevention, PEP and PrEP are needed not only in the major metropolitan areas, but in rural and sparsely populated towns and counties as well.

This book is about valuing these communities and presenting how best to provide the support they need to take care of themselves, to be able to overcome the barriers in their way, and to thrive. It lays out the case that rural health has both common and unique challenges when it comes to HIV and AIDS. This book is a useful tool to be utilized now and will stand as an ongoing resource to all of us who are working to prevent, reduce, and ultimately eliminate HIV and AIDS in rural America and beyond.

Disclaimer: The views expressed here are those of the author. No official endorsement by the U.S. Department of Health and Human Services or the National Institutes of Health is intended or should be inferred.

Paul Gaist, Ph.D., MPH

Coordinator and Health Scientist Administrator, Behavioral and Social Sciences Research Section, Office of AIDS Research, National Institutes of Health and Adjunct Professor, Department of Epidemiology, Johns Hopkins Bloomberg School of Public Health

Preface

Is there really a rural HIV epidemic?

This is a complex question. The vision of the National HIV/AIDS Strategy updated for 2020 is: "The United States will become a place where new HIV infections are rare, and when they do occur, every person, regardless of age, gender, race/ethnicity, sexual orientation, gender identity, or socioeconomic circumstances, will have unfettered access to high quality, life-extending care, free from stigma and discrimination" (White House Office of National AIDS Policy 2015). In addition, the Centers for Disease Control and Prevention (CDC) Fact Sheet titled "Today's HIV/AIDS Epidemic" indicates that prevention efforts have led to promising declines in new diagnoses and stabilization in new diagnoses among some high-risk populations such as gay and bisexual men and African-American women. Though overall HIV infection has decreased and HIV has become a treatable chronic disease, as many as 50,000 people still become newly infected annually. In addition to known risk behaviors, a range of social and economic factors situate some people at increased risk for HIV infection. HIV affects every corner of the United States. Data by region indicates the rate of infection is highest in the South (18.5 per 100,000 people), followed by the Northeast (14.2), West (11.2) and the Midwest (8.2) (Centers for Disease Control and Prevention 2016). The challenges and promising strategies of HIV/AIDS paint a different picture for urban verses rural America.

Small, charming and close-knit is the image of rural America. Yet in the fight against HIV/AIDS, rural communities face many of the same challenges as urban areas. But rural places everywhere concentrate many of the features that spread the HIV epidemic because they are small, close-knit communities. Individuals traveling back and forth from rural communities to urban centers add an additional dynamic to the rural setting. They are getting infected with new strains and may have more HIV mutations than once seen in rural communities. Moreover, the HIV/AIDS epidemic disproportionately affects southern rural poor and minority populations. Though rural areas have smaller numbers of HIV/AIDS cases, health system gaps due to healthcare provider shortages and vast distances mean not many specialized services are likely to be available. According to the Rural Center for AIDS/STD Prevention, rural life comes with the joy of a slower-paced life style, close-knit, supportive community, and wide-open spaces. On the other hand, some people feel trapped in rural communities due to inadequate educational opportunities, limited job opportunities, limited healthcare and social services, lack of public transportation, and isolation due to social stigma (Rural Center for AIDS/STD Prevention 2009, p. 1).

HIV/AIDS in Rural Communities: Research, Education, and Advocacy addresses many of the challenges and barriers to HIV/AIDS service delivery and care. Readers gain access to research, best practices and training resources for understanding HIV medicine and the latest on prevention, intervention, and care in rural settings. Moreover, the book presents ethical issues, cultural awareness, and advocacy models for service delivery and program implementation.

This book is an overview of HIV/AIDS in a unique context. The case examples offer a perspective on rural verses urban populations. Chapter authors present an overview of general access to health care then shift to the shortage of medical specialists trained in HIV prevention and care serving rural areas. Each chapter presents a compelling portrait of the challenges and promising strategies communities can adopt to build the HIV intervention and care continuum.

The history of HIV/AIDS over the past 30 plus years is a story that begins with the dramatic start of the epidemic in the United States in 1981 to present-day advances in prevention, treatment, and care. The Centers for Disease Control and Prevention (CDC) released its first Morbidity and Mortality Report on June 5, 1981. As early research struggled to understand the etiology, causes, and methods of transmission, the disease spread. Stigma and discrimination became widespread and deeply entrenched, causing people living with HIV/AIDS and even those who treated them immense suffering. This chapter offers a rear view mirror for understanding how the myths and misconceptions about HIV/AIDS drive stigma and discrimination, which still exist today, despite medical advances.

Advances in HIV Therapy is an overview of the change in treatment for HIV. Now a long-term, treatable, chronic disease, this chapter describes HIV medication; it describes why medications work and why they fail. Additionally, practical challenges are addressed such as state criminalization statues on HIV transmission, confidentiality, access to health care including pharmacy services and medication costs. The chapter offers solution-focused strategies for addressing barriers, finding support, and developing coping strategies such as good communication with medical providers.

"Treatment as Prevention (TasP)" is a phrase that people recognize in HIV prevention. This chapter reviews the literature on biomedical interventions that prevent HIV infection. As researchers, the authors recognize the limited data on these interventions in a rural context, but emphasize that TasP is an approach that works. With a vision to end HIV transmission, this chapter addresses biomedical, behavioral, and structural interventions that can be applied if resources are available and leadership is committed to adapt strategies to rural settings.

Ethical and legal issues in pediatric and adolescent HIV care require familiarity with federal laws, state laws, and consideration of confidentiality and disclosure dilemmas that health practitioners are likely to encounter. This chapter outlines considerations that are important in all settings, but emphasizes the relevance to rural settings where health disparities and limited resources are predominant.

HIV transmission from high-risk drug injection is associated with the surge in rural opioid use. Drug injection practices and high-risk sexual behaviors are risk factors for HIV transmission. This chapter compares the prevalence of HIV opioid use, treatment and harm reduction in rural versus urban settings as well as state and local efforts to control the spread of HIV and opioid use in rural communities. These efforts include improving access to substance abuse treatment and the use of harm reduction interventions.

Incorporating interviews from HIV positive African-American women who reside in the Deep South, this chapter presents the lessons learned and barriers still driving disparities for minorities living in the rural South. After 25 years as an HIV advocate and founder of a non-profit agency addressing the needs of African-American women living with HIV, this author shares insights on how race and ethnicity affect access to health care and other needed resources. With HIV infection growing fastest among African-American women through heterosexual exposure, this chapter offers strategies for intervention derived from the women most affected by the social determinants associated with higher rates of HIV/AIDS such as poor HIV literacy, lack of economic and educational opportunities, higher rates of other STDs, and social stigma.

The chapter on Black men who have sex with men (MSM) explores intersectional frameworks as a missing connection to effectively reduce HIV among marginalized communities. It describes intersectionality as a theoretical framework that examines how multiple socially constructed identities intersect at the level of individual experience. This dynamic impacts structural inequalities such as healthcare access. The author suggests the principles of intersectionality paired with minority stress theory are especially relevant for understanding the experiences of Black MSM.

The ten chapters included here address major contemporary issues for people affected by HIV/AIDS living in rural settings. Research, practical clinical approaches, and advocacy models attest to hopeful strategies for HIV prevention, intervention, and care in rural communities despite critical issues and limited resources. All the authors included in this book agree that healthcare patients and providers will benefit greatly from research and practices that incorporate rural people's unique perspectives.

Statesboro, USA   Fayth M. Parks
Atlanta, USA   Gregory S. Felzien
Los Angeles, USA   Sally Jue

References

Centers for Disease Control and Prevention. (2016, August). CDC fact sheet: Today's HIV/AIDS epidemic. Retrieved from https://www.cdc.gov/nchhstp/newsroom/docs/factsheets/todaysepidemic-508.pdf

Rural Center for AIDS/STD Prevention. (2009). Fact sheet: HIV/AIDS in rural America: Challenges and promising strategies. Retrieved from http://www.indiana.edu/~aids/publications/fact-sheets/

White House Office of National AIDS Policy. (2015, July). National HIV/AIDS Strategy for the United States: 2020. Washington, DC: White House Office of National AIDS Policy. Retrieved from https://www.aids.gov/federal-resources/national-hiv-aids-strategy/nhas-update/index.html

Contents

Editors and Contributors

About the Editors

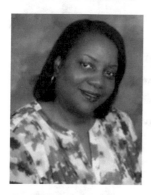

Fayth M. Parks, Ph.D. is an Associate Professor and licensed psychologist in the Department of Leadership, Technology, and Human Development at Georgia Southern University. From 2010 to 2012, she was an HIV/AIDS trainer through the American Psychological Association's (APA) HIV Office for Psychology Education (HOPE). In 2012, Dr. Parks was inspired by the HOPE training program to found the Rural HIV Research and Training Conference held annually in Savannah, Georgia. She serves on the Steering Committee for the Southeast AIDS Education and Training Center (SE AETC). She is also chair of the APA Ad Hoc Committee on Psychology and AIDS (COPA). Dr. Parks has written and lectured extensively on cultural diversity in health and illness, healing practices, and traditional medicine. In 2009, she was the David B. Larson Fellow in Health and Spirituality at The John W. Kluge Center of the Library of Congress.

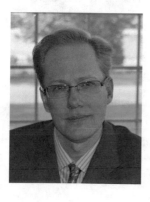

Gregory S. Felzien, MD, AAHIVS is board certified in both internal medicine and infectious diseases and also certified as an American Academy of HIV specialist. He is a medical advisor within the Georgia Department of Public Health's Division of Health Protection/IDI-HIV. As part of this position, Dr. Felzien continues to care for and focus on the needs of rural HIV positive individuals throughout the state. Dr. Felzien practices infectious disease medicine with an emphasis on HIV, tuberculosis, and hepatitis. He is actively involved in the rural community through coordinating HIV awareness and education and writing and speaking at the local, state, and national levels. He is also as a member of the provider advisory board for the CDC's HIV medical monitoring program and Steering Committee for the Southeast AIDS Education and Training Center (SE AETC).

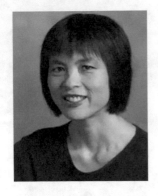

Sally Jue, MSW is a former manager at AIDS Project Los Angeles, where she created and managed one of the first HIV mental health programs in the United States. She and her staff created innovative clinical treatment programs for clients with co-occurring disorders as well as volunteer peer support programs. In addition to overseeing staff, peer, professional volunteers, and interns, Ms. Jue was also active in developing partnerships that brought together different organizations and communities to advocate for improved access to services for people affected by HIV. Ms. Jue is a founder and former chair of the LA County HIV Asian Pacific Caucus, a former consultant for the SAMHSA Mental Health HIV Services Collaborative, and former appointee to the LA County Department of Health Services' Cultural and Linguistic Competency Standards Work Group.

Contributors

Barbara J. Blake WellStar School of Nursing, Kennesaw State University, Kennesaw, GA, USA

Neal A. Carnes Georgia State University, Atlanta, USA

Jarvis W. Carter Jr. Division of HIV/AIDS Prevention/Prevention Research Branch, Centers for Disease Control & Prevention, Atlanta, GA, USA

Tiffany Chenneville Department of Psychology, University of South Florida St. Petersburg, St. Petersburg, FL, USA

Cherie Drenzek Division of Health Protection, Georgia Department of Public Health, Atlanta, GA, USA

Gregory S. Felzien Georgia Department of Public Health, Division of Health Protection/IDI-HIV, Atlanta, GA, USA

Nathan Hansen Department of Health Promotion and Behavior, University of Georgia College of Public Health, Athens, GA, USA

Jordan Helms Emory University—Rollins School of Public Health, Atlanta, USA

Susan Hrostowski Social Work, The University of Southern Mississippi, Hattiesburg, MS, USA

Brian Huylebroeck HIV Epidemiology, Georgia Department of Public Health, Atlanta, GA, USA

Jane Kelly HIV Epidemiology, Georgia Department of Public Health, Atlanta, GA, USA

Danielle Lambert Department of Health Promotion and Behavior, University of Georgia College of Public Health, Athens, GA, USA

Carolyn Lauckner Department of Health Promotion and Behavior, University of Georgia College of Public Health, Athens, GA, USA

Jennifer D. Lenardson Maine Rural Health Research Center, University of Southern Maine, Portland, ME, USA

John Malone Georgia Department of Public Health, Atlanta, USA

Anne O. Odusanya Department of Community Health Behavior and Education, Jiann-Ping Hsu College of Public Health, Georgia Southern University, Statesboro, GA, USA

Deepali Rane DOCS Operations CPC, DOCS Global, Atlanta, GA, USA

Anne Marie Schipani-McLaughlin Department of Health Promotion and Behavior, University of Georgia College of Public Health, Athens, GA, USA

Stacy W. Smallwood Department of Community Health Behavior & Education, Jiann-Ping Hsu College of Public Health, Georgia Southern University, Statesboro, GA, USA

Mary Lindsey Smith Maine Rural Health Research Center, University of Southern Maine, Portland, ME, USA

Gloria Ann Jones Taylor WellStar School of Nursing, Kennesaw State University, Kennesaw, GA, USA

Pascale Wortley HIV Epidemiology, Georgia Department of Public Health, Atlanta, GA, USA

Catherine Wyatt-Morley Women On Maintaining Education and Nutrition, Nashville, TN, USA

Part I
HIV and Rural Communities

Chapter 1
Case Study: Georgia's Rural Versus Non-rural Populations

Jane Kelly, Deepali Rane, Brian Huylebroeck, Pascale Wortley and Cherie Drenzek

Background

In 2014, Georgia's estimated population was 10,097,343, with 1,771,244 people living in rural Georgia. According to the Georgia State Office of Rural Health (SORH), rural Georgians are more likely to be underinsured or uninsured, more likely to suffer from heart disease, diabetes and cancer, and more likely to live in an area with a shortage of mental health, dental, and medical primary care providers than their urban counterparts (SORH, 2015). An estimated 25.3% of rural Georgians live in poverty, in contrast to 17.7% poverty rate in urban areas (Rural Health Information Hub, 2015). In a 2015 poll of rural Georgians on healthcare needs, more than three-fourths reported a moderate (49.5%) or serious/extreme (27.7%) shortage of healthcare providers. Additionally, 18% of rural Georgians noted lack of

J. Kelly (✉) · B. Huylebroeck · P. Wortley
HIV Epidemiology, Georgia Department of Public Health, 2 Peachtree Street, NW, Suite 14-420, Atlanta, GA 30303, USA
e-mail: jane.kelly@dph.ga.gov

B. Huylebroeck
e-mail: Brian.Huylebroeck@dph.ga.gov

P. Wortley
e-mail: pascale.wortley@dph.ga.gov

D. Rane
DOCS Operations CPC, DOCS Global, 2207 Lakeshore Crossing NE, Atlanta, GA 30324, USA
e-mail: deepali.rane@docsglobal.com

C. Drenzek
Division of Health Protection, Georgia Department of Public Health, 2 Peachtree Street, NW, 14th Floor, 14-450, Atlanta, GA 30303, USA
e-mail: cherie.drenzek@dph.ga.gov

© Springer International Publishing AG 2017
F.M. Parks et al. (eds.), *HIV/AIDS in Rural Communities*,
DOI 10.1007/978-3-319-56239-1_1

transportation as a barrier to accessing medical care (Georgia Healthcare Foundation, 2015).

Against this backdrop of general need, the availability of medical specialists trained in HIV prevention and care serving rural areas is even more acute. With the advent of effective antiretroviral therapy (ART), HIV has become a treatable chronic disease. Nationally, survival after an HIV diagnosis was estimated to be 29 years in 2011, with substantially lower average survival for those with AIDS at diagnosis (24 years) and injection drug users (20 and 21 years for male and female IDU, respectively) (Siddiqi, Hall, Hu, & Song, 2016). However, HIV care is complicated by late diagnosis, variable access to care, comorbid conditions that hinder treatment, stigma, and discrimination. Persons living with HIV (PLWH) have known higher levels of poverty, mental illness (both mood and thought disorders), and alcohol and nonprescription drug or prescription drug abuse (CDC, 2011). Nonurban areas are challenged to provide not only HIV medical care but also support services, e.g., mental health and substance abuse counseling, housing, and social assistance.

The shortage of healthcare providers in rural areas who are trained and willing to treat PLWH presents a serious challenge. While services provided through the Ryan White program offer care for uninsured or underinsured PLWH, nationwide 95% of rural counties lacked a Ryan White medical provider, versus 69% of urban counties in 2013 (Vyavaharkar, et al., 2013). In Georgia, aside from Ryan White Part A clinics in urban Atlanta, there are only 20 full-time Part B clinics serving the rest of the state; nine of which provide care for 8–16 counties. Three provide case management and AIDS Drug Assistance Program (ADAP) services only, with no clinical services onsite. Ten satellite clinics provide additional outreach but are open intermittently, e.g., six times annually, or varying days and hours depending on the week of the month, or by appointment only. One provides pediatric HIV care one-half day twice per week. Only one offers services for a half day on Saturday; three are open to 7PM one day a week. Access to care is a challenge for PLWH in rural areas (Georgia DPH, 2014b).

In 2014, Georgia was ranked fifth in the nation for HIV prevalence, with 53,218 PLWH, 53% of whom had Stage 3 disease or AIDS. Of the 4790 new diagnoses made in Georgia in 2013–2014 for whom we have CD4 counts within 12 months of diagnosis, 29% were late testers, i.e., they had already developed AIDS (CD4 < 200) at or within 12 months of diagnosis, implying that they had likely been living with HIV for at least 8 years. Over two-thirds (70%) of PLWH in 2014 resided in the Atlanta Metropolitan Statistical Area (MSA) with substantial numbers of PLWH in Augusta, Savannah, Columbus, and other urban areas (Georgia DPH, 2014b).

The HIV Care Continuum

Name-based HIV case reporting became law in Georgia in 2004. In addition, all laboratories licensed in the state are required to submit HIV-related laboratory reports, including undetectable viral load results (VL), to the Georgia Department of Public Health (DPH) HIV/AIDS Epidemiology section. Case report forms and laboratory results are uploaded into the enhanced HIV/AIDS Reporting System (eHARS). From this database, we can construct analyses of the HIV care continuum, e.g., the number and proportion of persons linked to care, retained in care, and achieving viral suppression (VS) using reported laboratory test data. We constructed the HIV Care Continuum for Georgia for 2014 with these criteria:

- Adults and adolescents aged 13 and older diagnosed with HIV by 12/31/2013, living as of 12/31/2014
- Current address within Georgia
- Linked to care within 30 days = CD4 or VL drawn within 30 days of diagnosis for new diagnoses in 2014
- Any care: ≥ 1 CD4 or VL reported in 2014
- Retained in care: ≥ 2 CD4 or VL reported at least 3 months apart in 2014
- Viral suppression (VS): VL < 200 for the most recent VL in 2014*
  * This epidemiologic definition for VS is consistent with the care continuum literature, and is not the same as the clinical definition of undetectable viral load.

Among new diagnoses in Georgia in 2014 overall, 75% were linked to care within 30 days of their first visit. Among all persons living with HIV in Georgia, 61% had at least one CD4 or VL laboratory test done in 2014, which we define here as having received "Any Care", 48% were "Retained in Care", and 45% achieved VS (Fig. 1.1).

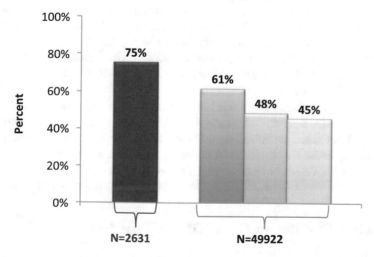

Fig. 1.1 HIV Care Continuum for Georgia, 2014

Stratification by demographics has identified disparities by race, age, sex, and transmission category nationally and in Georgia (CDC, 2014; Georgia DPH, 2014b). Additional analysis by geographic location reflects another level of disparity.

HIV Care Continuum by Eligible Metropolitan Area (EMA) Versus Non-EMA

The Ryan White program provides HIV clinical care and services for PLWH. Ryan White is divided into several parts. Part A provides funding for Eligible Metropolitan Areas (EMAs), which are defined as population centers of at least 50,000 people that have reported 2000 or more AIDS cases in the most recent 5 years. For the purposes of monitoring and addressing the HIV care needs of the state, Georgia can be divided into the Atlanta EMA (Bartow, Paulding, Carroll, Coweta, Fayette, Spalding, Henry, Newton, Rockdale, Gwinnett, Walton, Barrow, Forsyth, Cherokee, Pickens, DeKalb, Fulton, Clayton, Cobb and Douglas counties) and the non-EMA (all other counties in Georgia) (Fig. 1.2).

The majority (34,593/49,922 or 69%) of PLWH in Georgia have a current address in the Atlanta EMA. This address is referred to as their "current" address, though it may be several years old, and may not represent their true current address if they moved and have not had a lab result reported containing an updated address.

The proportions linked to care, and virally suppressed (overall and among those retained), were lower among persons residing in non-EMA counties than in the EMA in almost every stratum (HIV Care Continuum report, Georgia DPH, 2014). While the proportion retained in care was significantly higher ($p < 0.05$) among persons living in non-EMA counties compared to the EMA overall, the proportion of PLWH achieving VS was significantly higher in the EMA for all subgroups except IDU and MSM/IDU. Although not statistically significant, the substantial difference in VS for PLWH aged 13–19 years living in the EMA (57%) compared to non-EMA (39%) is concerning.

VS among those retained in care was lower overall and in many strata for PLWH residing in non-EMA than those residing in EMA counties in Georgia. Although differences did not reach statistical significance, there was a consistent pattern of lower VS among residents of non-EMA counties, and there was no instance where the proportion with VS was higher among PLWH residing in non-EMA counties.

Rural-Urban Continuum Codes (RUCC) Analysis

To look beyond the Atlanta EMA/non-EMA comparison, we used the 2013 Rural-Urban Continuum Codes (RUCC), which classify each county in the United States into one of nine categories by degree of urbanization and adjacency to a

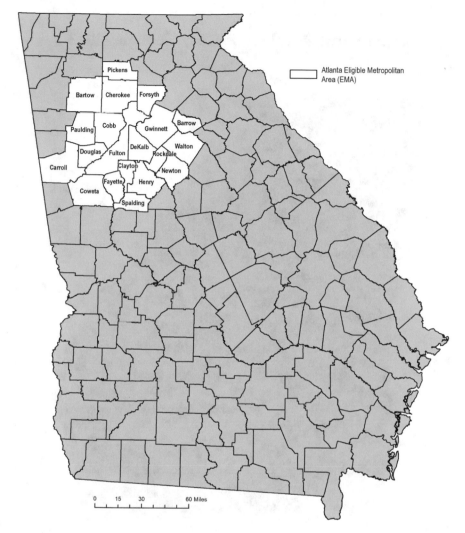

Fig. 1.2 Atlanta Eligible Metropolitan Areas (EMA) and non-EMA areas, Georgia, 2014

metropolitan area (USDA, 2013). We dichotomized these nine classifications into metropolitan and nonmetropolitan by combining three metropolitan and six non-metropolitan categories. The metropolitan areas in this analysis included all counties in metropolitan areas, and the non-metropolitan areas included all other counties of Georgia (Fig. 1.3). In this analysis, 87% (42,655/48,957) PLWH in Georgia in 2014 lived in metropolitan areas, 11% (5008/48,957) in non-metropolitan areas, with current address information missing for 3% (1294/48,957). For the purpose of this analysis, metropolitan counties will be referred to as urban, and non-metropolitan counties as rural.

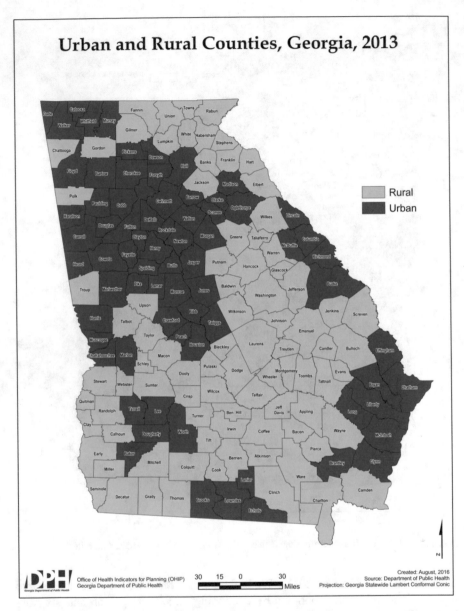

Fig. 1.3 Georgia urban and rural counties by Rural-Urban Continuum Codes (RUCC), 2013

Using the same definitions and inclusion criteria as was used in the EMA and non-EMA analysis, we assessed the HIV care continuum and association with individual demographic characteristics across urban and rural areas (Table 1.1).

Overall, receipt of any care, and retention in care were higher in rural counties than in urban counties, and the proportion achieving VS was similar in urban and

Table 1.1 Linkage; any care, retained in care, VS, and VS among those retained in care, Georgia, 2014

	Linked to care N (%)		Any care N (%)		Retained in care N (%)		Viral suppression (VS) N (%)		VS among retained N (%)	
	Rural	Urban	Rural	Urban	Rural	Urban	Rural	Urban	Rural	Urban
Overall	71% (212)	74% (2,379)	65% (5008)	62% (42,655)	54% (5008)	49% (42,655)	45% (5008)	47% (42,655)	75% (2709)	82% (20,733)
Sex										
Male	69% (157)	74% (1916)	65% (3344)	61% (32,327)	54% (3344)	48% (32,327)	46% (3344)	47% (32,327)	76% (1798)	83% (15,601)
Female	74% (54)	73% (456)	65% (1660)	63% (10,248)	55% (1660)	50% (10,248)	44% (1660)	46% (10,248)	73% (911)	79% (5126)
Race/Ethnicity										
Black	65% (141)	71% (1558)	66% (3322)	62% (28,519)	55% (3322)	47% (28,519)	45% (3322)	44% (28,519)	73% (1837)	78% (13,616)
Hispanic/Latino	N < 10	70% (129)	54% (256)	58% (2495)	48% (256)	49% (2495)	39% (256)	47% (2495)	78% (120)	85% (1232)
White	77% (36)	81% (317)	66% (1051)	63% (8331)	54% (1051)	51% (8331)	50% (1051)	53% (8331)	81% (580)	89% (4263)
Transmission category										
MSM	70% (115)	72% (1456)	67% (2243)	63% (25,283)	56% (2243)	49% (25,283)	48% (2243)	48% (25,283)	76% (1254)	83% (12,483)
IDU	69% (10)	78% (78)	61% (522)	54% (3215)	50% (522)	43% (3215)	43% (522)	40% (3215)	76% (262)	80% (1386)
MSM/IDU	N < 10	72% (39)	69% (188)	57% (1966)	55% (188)	46% (1966)	49% (188)	41% (1966)	78% (104)	79% (902)
HET	70% (64)	74% (487)	66% (1833)	64% (10,151)	56% (1833)	51% (10,151)	45% (1833)	47% (10,151)	74% (1033)	79% (5156)

(continued)

Table 1.1 (continued)

	Linked to care N (%)		Any care N (%)		Retained in care N (%)		Viral suppression (VS) N (%)		VS among retained N (%)	
	Rural	Urban	Rural	Urban	Rural	Urban	Rural	Urban	Rural	Urban
Age (in years)										
13–24	61% (57)	67% (540)	63% (186)	**66% (1535)**	52% (186)	49% (1535)	37% (186)	42% (1535)	64% (96)	72% (745)
25–34	**77% (61)**	**73% (737)**	64% (792)	60% (7647)	**51% (792)**	**45% (7647)**	41% (792)	39% (7647)	71% (402)	72% (3407)
35–44	77% (44)	78% (473)	64% (1165)	**61% (10,088)**	**53% (1165)**	**47% (10,088)**	46% (1165)	46% (10,088)	77% (615)	81% (4785)
45–54	**67% (27)**	**77% (401)**	67% (1637)	**62% (14,171)**	**57% (1637)**	**50% (14,171)**	48% (1637)	49% (14,171)	**77% (931)**	**84% (7161)**
55 and older	74% (23)	79% (228)	**63% (1228)**	61% (9214)	54% (1228)	50% (9214)	45% (1228)	50% (9214)	74% (665)	**88% (4635)**

Proportional differences that are statistically significant with $P < 0.05$ are indicated by bold font

MSM men who have sex with men; *IDU* injection drug user; *HET* heterosexual

Sample Size = 48,957 total, 42,655 Metro, 5008 non-Metro, 1294 Unknown address

Source Georgia enhanced HIV/AIDS Reporting System (eHARS), 2016

rural counties. Statistically significant differences in VS were seen only for MSM/IDU (49% rural, 41% urban) and for Hispanics (39% rural, 47% urban). The proportion virally suppressed among those retained in care was higher overall among persons in urban counties, with statistically significant differences for multiple subgroups. This highlights the importance of considering not only VS, for which there was no consistent difference between most rural and urban populations, but also VS among those retained in care. Assessing VS among persons retained in care demonstrates that disparities in VS are not simply a function of access to and retention in care, but reflect other factors influencing antiretroviral therapy (ART) use and adherence, including clinicians' failure to follow clinical practice guidelines and patients' missing ART doses. VS among persons retained in care was significantly higher in urban Georgia overall and for males, Blacks, Whites, MSM, and persons aged 45 years and older. There were no subgroups in which the proportion virally suppressed among those retained in care was significantly higher among residents of rural areas than among residents of urban areas.

Limitations

People who have out-migrated to, or seek care in other states, will appear as out of care with no VS, potentially resulting in underestimation of VS. This could impact the results if out-migration disproportionately affects urban or rural residents, but we are unable to measure this. People living in a rural area may receive treatment in an urban area, complicating understanding of relationship between residence and care. Our definition of rural includes all counties that were not part of a metropolitan statistical area, which includes residents of smaller cities. As a result, generalizability to more rural areas is limited.

HIV Outcomes in Rural Georgia

What are some of the factors interfering with achieving VS among persons retained in care in rural Georgia? Despite possibly greater challenges of distance to a healthcare provider, and limited public transportation, PLWH in rural areas often had greater retention in care than those in urban areas. Yet VS among persons retained in care was lower. Possible explanations include less frequent prescribing of antiretroviral therapy (ART) and/or decreased ART adherence, perhaps with societal, patient-level, healthcare system-level influencing factors.

Racial Disparity

A lower proportion of Black PLWH achieved VS compared to Whites in both rural and urban areas. Only in rural areas was the proportion of Hispanic/Latinos achieving VS and retention in care lower than among Blacks, possibly a function of more transient agricultural worker status among Hispanic/Latinos in these areas, potentially combined with less awareness of Ryan White clinics. Nevertheless, among those retained in care, a lower proportion of Blacks achieved VS than Hispanic/Latinos and Whites in both urban and rural areas. Possible reasons may include Black/White racial differences in physiological responses to medications, as has been found with anti-hypertensive medications, thus impacting outcomes (Gupta, 2010). However, no biological factors such as differential drug absorption, metabolism, or tolerance among US Blacks compared to Whites have been found for various ART regimens, leading researchers to conclude that lower VS is driven by social factors (Ribaudo, 2013).

Stigma

In addition to fewer support services and poverty, one must consider the psycho-dynamics of living in rural Georgia with HIV. In general, the culture in the rural South is one of greater religiosity, homophobia, and negative attitudes towards PLWH, especially in Black communities (Visser, Kershaw, Matkin, & Forsyth, 2008; Foster, 2007). Stigma inhibits HIV status disclosure and increases fear of confidentiality breach, thus isolating the person living with HIV, and acts as a barrier to care (Southern AIDS Coalition, 2008; Heckman et al., 1998). Internalized stigma, leading to shame and decreased self-worth, and lack of perceived social support negatively affect ART adherence (Langebeek et al., 2014; Turan et al., 2016).

Internalized Homonegativity

Homonegativity (the extent to which MSM have internalized society's negative attitudes towards same-sex attraction and relationships) affects sexual risk behaviors. An analysis of Houston National HIV Behavioral Surveillance data found that Black MSM had higher homonegativity scores than Whites or Latinos (27% vs. 21% and 23% for Blacks, Whites and Hispanic/Latinos respectively) ($p = 0.01$) (Padgett, Risser, Khuwaja, Lopez, & Troisi, 2015). Blacks living in the non-EMA counties had the lowest proportion of VS among those retained, which is possibly related to internalized homonegativity and stigma of living with HIV in rural Georgia.

Denial and Social Isolation

Loneliness among rural MSM was associated with increased risk behaviors, e.g., condomless sex with a partner of unknown HIV status (Hubach et al., 2015). Geographic isolation of men who have sex with men (MSM), the highest risk group for HIV infection, creates additional barriers to HIV prevention and care. Rural MSM are less likely to think HIV is a problem where they live (Williams, Bowen, & Horvath, 2005; Rosser, 2001), are less likely to seek HIV testing (Hall, Li, & McKenna, 2005), have fewer opportunities to socialize with other MSM, and are more likely to seek out casual sex partners at truck stops (Rosser, 2001) than their urban counterparts.

Injection Drug Use

Injection drug use (IDU) contributes a small proportion of new HIV diagnoses in Georgia, but rural areas may be at increased risk of outbreaks associated with injection drug use similar to the 2015 outbreak in Scott County, Indiana associated with changing patterns of opioid use (CDC, 2015). An analysis of indicator variables highly associated with IDU identified 220 counties in 26 states as vulnerable for a similar HIV outbreak, including several rural counties in north Georgia (Van Handel et al., 2016). The stereotype of IDU as an urban problem fails to recognize that rural areas suffer from decreased access to substance abuse treatment and harm reduction (e.g., syringe exchange) programs, lower risk awareness, lower education levels, and higher poverty and unemployment, leaving a population vulnerable for rapid HIV spread.

HIV Workforce

The diminishing HIV workforce adds to the challenges in meeting the 2020 National HIV/AIDS Strategy objectives. This disparity of decreasing numbers of HIV providers in the face of increasing numbers of PLWH is a crisis not only for Georgia, but nationwide, arguably affecting rural areas more because of a paucity of infectious disease specialists. The current HIV medical workforce is largely composed of the first generation of HIV medical providers who entered the field more than 20 years ago. According to the Human Resource and Services Administration (HRSA) estimates, there is already a shortage of 7000 primary care physicians in underserved areas (HRSA, 2010a, b). A 2008 survey of Ryan White HIV/AIDS Program-funded clinics noted

- 51% of clinics reported up to a 25% increase in caseloads.
- 20% reported more than a 25% increase in caseloads in the previous 3 years.

- 69% of clinics reported difficulty recruiting HIV clinicians and cited reimbursement and lack of providers as leading causes (HRSA, 2010a, b).

Without appropriate workforce capacity building, clinics that serve PLWH may be forced to reduce services, cut back clinic hours, or close facilities entirely. Financial disincentives are an ever-growing issue in attracting providers to the field of HIV (HIV Specialist, 2016). The proportion of medical graduates in Georgia with debts over $20,000 has increased from 13.4% in 2008 to 42.0% in 2014 (GBPW, 2014). Traditionally, specialties with reimbursement for procedures (e.g., cardiology, gastroenterology) make higher salaries than those paid for non-procedural cognitive services (primary care, infectious disease). Considering the lesser remuneration for HIV care, this debt burden suggests another challenge to developing an adequate HIV workforce, especially in rural areas.

Within the state of Georgia, the Georgia Board for Physician Workforce (GBPW) June 2013 report highlights include these estimates:

- Between 2000 and 2010, the population in Georgia increased 18.3%.
- Between 2007 and 2014, the diagnosed HIV population in Georgia increased 58% from 33,719 to 53,230 (as per Georgia DPH HIV surveillance data).
- In 2010 Georgia ranked 41st nationally in the number of primary care physicians per 100,000.
- The number of physicians per 100,000 in clinical specialties likely to deliver HIV care remained fairly flat during the years 1998–2010 in Georgia (Table 1.2).
- More than half (52.3%) of all Georgia's physicians are located in five Primary Care Service Areas (PCSAs) that represent 37% of the state's population. These PCSAs are in urban areas of Atlanta and Augusta (Fulton, DeKalb, Columbia, Lincoln, Richmond, Cobb, Paulding, and Gwinnett Counties).
- Almost one-third (32.7%) of the workforce is not accepting new Medicaid patients.
- In 2010, more than half (52.7%) of the physician workforce was aged 50 years and older, compared to a third (33.8%) in 2000.
- 10.5% of Georgia's physician workforce indicated they plan to retire in the next 5 years (GBPW, 2013).

According to the Association of American Medical Colleges (AAMC), Georgia Physician Workforce Profile, the number of practicing physicians in Georgia demonstrates underrepresentation of primary care and infectious disease clinicians (AAMC, 2015):

Table 1.2 Georgia physicians by specialty and rate per 100,000, 1998–2010

Specialty	1998	2000	2002	2004	2006	2008	2010
Family/General practice	26.52	26.18	25.36	26.40	26.24	26.47	27.14
Infectious disease	1.32	1.20	1.56	1.71	2.25	2.21	2.24
Internal medicine	25.79	27.66	29.30	30.53	27.12	26.22	27.80
Public health	1.52	1.16	0.80	0.86	1.25	1.24	0.54

Specialty	Total Active Physicians
All Specialties	22,303
Family Medicine/General Practice	2781
Infectious Disease	260 (Majority in Fulton, DeKalb and Richmond Counties)
Internal Medicine	3153

What are the future prospects for an increased HIV workforce in Georgia to meet increasing need? The shortage of Infectious Disease physicians in the face of an increasing HIV patient population challenges the approach of HIV care delivered predominantly by specialists rather than primary care clinicians, and compels us to change our healthcare model for HIV (HealthHIV, 2012). Concerns about quality of care offered by providers with small HIV caseloads must be addressed (HIV Specialist, 2016). HIV care indicators, such as proportion of patients achieving VS, was lower for New York clinicians prescribing ART for <20 patients in 2009 than for more experienced providers in established HIV care centers (O'Neill et al., 2015). A similar situation in Georgia could explain the lower VS among those retained in care in rural versus urban areas.

Solutions

Extending the Reach of HIV Professionals

The current healthcare system in Georgia does not have the capacity to absorb the influx of new patients if all HIV-positive clients were linked to care. TeleMedicine (TeleHealth) is an underutilized resource for providing specialty care to resource-poor, typically rural, areas. Yet, by using urban providers, TeleMedicine adds an additional burden to an already strained urban system. There are simply not enough HIV care providers at present to care for all of the PLWH throughout Georgia, a situation that is likely true nationally as well. Free online continuing medical education programs such as the International Antiviral Society-USA (IAS-USA) Cases on the Web (IAS-USA, 2016) and educational curriculum "Expanding the HIV Provider Base: Preparing Clinicians for HIV Care" developed by the AAHIVM, California Academy of Family Physicians and Medscape Education (Medscape, 2014) help, but do not substitute for hands-on training experiences, and must be continually updated. AIDS Education and Training Centers (AETC) provide online educational programs, phone consultation, didactic and clinical educational training opportunities, including those targeting nurse practitioners physician assistants (AETC, 2016). Local efforts to increase workforce capacity include the 2-year Los Angeles County HIV Public Health Fellowship (LACHPHF) for primary care clinicians. Funded by a 5-year $7.5 million grant, the training is slated to begin in 2016 and anticipated to enroll 10–18 physicians (LACHPHF, 2016). In addition to providing training, the fellowship offers loan repayment grants of up to $50,000/year for 3 years for those working in under-served communities. The Family Medicine Residency of Idaho HIV Primary Care Fellowship offers a 12-month post-residency training. Increasingly, Family Medicine residencies offer Areas of Concentration (AOC) that allow residents to tailor their clinical experience, such as the Lancaster Family Medicine Program AOC in HIV primary care (Lancaster, 2016). University of California, San Francisco (UCSF) and Wooster, MA offer similar HIV AOCs. The results of these individual program efforts may be small; e.g., as of March 2016, the Lancaster Program has trained 11 residents who have become certified by AAHIVM as HIV specialists, but the program represents a model for increasing capacity of rural HIV care. Extending the reach of HIV professionals must include increased utilization of advanced practice nurses, physician assistants, pharmacists, registered nurses, and social workers in a team approach (HIV Specialist, 2016).

Targeted Partner Services

Limited capacity and resources prevent Georgia from providing partner services for all PLWH in the state, and because rural areas have a lower HIV prevalence, generalized approaches to increasing HIV testing to find the undiagnosed are not optimal. Targeted strategies that prioritize referring new infections and sentinel events (e.g., established HIV infection with a new STI) for partner services was demonstrated to have a higher yield for identifying new infections in low-prevalence rural New Mexico (Gans & Murph, 2015) and may offer an effective approach in other rural areas.

Social Media

The increasing role of social media, phone apps, and online services offers not only an opportunity to reach rural populations with HIV prevention and treatment messages (Badal, Stryker, DeLuca, & Purcell, 2015), but also a mechanism to relieve the social isolation PLWH often feel, especially in rural areas. A study of the effectiveness of ads on dating/hookup websites demonstrated that MSM will "click through" to access HIV prevention messages while looking for sexual partners via mobile apps (DeLuca, Badal, Stryker, Boudewyns, Stine, & Purcell, 2015). Focus groups with young (aged 16–21 years) MSM emphasized the homonegativity, fear of "outing", and stigma they experience, and described social media networks as a supportive way to "hang out" with an online same-sex community (Sitron, Hawkins, Schlupp, Franklin, Johnson, & Brady, 2015). Leveraging online community connectedness for rural young MSM can be an important tool in reducing the social isolation and fear of disclosure that hinder safer sex behaviors, such as negotiating sexual interactions. The healthMpowerment program, a mobile phone app intervention, delivers information, individualized feedback, entertainment, and a social networking platform providing peer support for HIV-positive and negative young (aged 18–30 years) black MSM (Hightow-Weidman, Muessig, Soni, Pike, Kirschke-Schwartz, & LeGrand, 2015). Such a phone app intervention can potentially reach rural young Black MSM in nontraditional ways to assist with retention in care, address ART adherence issues, and provide a peer community connection.

Faith-Based Institution Outreach

Increasingly, programs through faith-based institutions, especially churches with a predominantly Black congregation, have attempted to address stigma. An interactive, culturally based, anti-stigma campaign pilot tested in Black Churches in rural Alabama shows promise (Aholou, Payne-Foster, Cooks, Sutton, & Gaskins, 2015).

Conclusion

While it is encouraging that rural PLWH appear to be retained in HIV care at least as well, and sometimes with a higher proportion, than their urban counterparts, it is disturbing that fewer of those in care and living in rural areas achieve VS. Meeting the needs of an increasing number of PLWH in the face of a diminishing HIV workforce is a daunting task in Georgia, and likely to be exacerbated in rural areas in coming years, unless there is a paradigm shift in our pubic health and medical team model for HIV prevention and care.

References

Aholou, T., Payne-Foster, P., Cooks, E., Sutton, M., & Gaskins, S. (2015, December). Healing through FAITHH: Developing an HIV Stigma Reduction Intervention. *Abstracts of the 2016 National HIV Prevention Conference*. Atlanta, GA. Abstract 1414.

AIDS Education and Training Center Program. (2016). *Expanding HIV Training into Graduate/Health Profession Education*. (Internet) http://www.aidsetc.org/special-initiatives/health-professions. Accessed June 17, 2016.

Association of American Medical Colleges. (2015). *2015 State Data Book Snapshots, Georgia Profile*. (Internet) https://www.aamc.org/download/447164/data/georgiaprofile.pdf. Accessed June 17, 2016.

Badal, H., Stryker, J., DeLuca, N., & Purcell, D. (2015, December). Swipe left: Dating/Hookup website and app use among men who have sex with men. *Abstracts of the 2016 National HIV Prevention Conference*. Atlanta, GA. Abstract 1660.

Centers for Disease Control and Prevention (CDC). (2011). Clinical and behavioral characteristics of adults receiving medical care for HIV infection—Medical Monitoring Project, United States, 2007. *MMWR, 60*(SS-11):1–11.

Centers for Disease Control and Prevention (CDC). (2014). Vital signs: HIV diagnosis, care, and treatment among persons living with HIV—United States, 2011. *MMWR, 63*(47), 1113–1117.

Centers for Disease Control and Prevention (CDC). (2015). Community outbreak of HIV infection linked to injection drug use of oxymorphone—Indiana, 2015. *MMWR,* May 1, 2015, *64*(16), 443–444.

DeLuca, N., Badal, H., Stryker, J., Boudewyns, V., Stine, A., & Purcell, D. (2015, December). Sex sells: Utilizing effective digital channels to reach men who have sex with men with HIV testing and prevention messages. *Abstracts of the 2016 National HIV Prevention Conference.* Atlanta, GA. Abstract 1762.

Family Medicine Residency of Idaho HIV Primary Care Fellowship. (Internet) http://www.fmridaho.org/residency/fellowship/hiv-primary-care/

Foster, P. H. (2007). Use of stigma, fear, and denial in development of a framework for prevention of HIV/AIDS in rural African American communities. *Family & Community Health, 30*(4), 318–327.

Gans, A., & Murph, J. (2015, December). HIV case finding using partner services in a low prevalence state. *Abstracts of the 2016 National HIV Prevention Conference.* Atlanta, GA. Abstract 2410.

Georgia Board for Physician Workforce. (2013, December). *Physician and Physician Assistant Professions Data Book 2010/2011.* (Internet) https://gbpw.georgia.gov/sites/gbpw.georgia.gov/files/related_files/document/2010-2011%20Data%20Book%20%289.19.14%29.pdf. Accessed June 17, 2016.

Georgia Board of Physician Workforce. (2014, June). *Graduate Medical Education Survey Reports.* (Internet) https://gbpw.georgia.gov/sites/gbpw.georgia.gov/files/related_files/site_page/GME%20Exit%20Survey%202014.pdf%20%28Final%2012-15-14%29.pdf. Accessed June 17, 2016.

Georgia Department of Public Health, HIV/AIDS Epidemiology Section. (2014a). *HIV Care Continuum, Georgia.* (Internet) http://dph.georgia.gov/hiv-care-continuum Accessed June 16, 2016.

Georgia Department of Public Health, HIV/AIDS Epidemiology Section. (2014b). *HIV surveillance summary.* (Internet) https://dph.georgia.gov/data-fact-sheet-summaries. Accessed June 16, 2016.

Georgia Department of Public Health, HIV/AIDS Care Services. *Statewide HIV care and service providers.* (Internet) https://dph.georgia.gov/statewide-hiv-care-service-providers. Accessed June 6, 2016.

Georgia Healthcare Foundation. (2015). *Health voices—Rural health and health care in Georgia: 2015 Georgia poll results.* (Internet) http://www.healthcaregeorgia.org/uploads/publications/HealthVoices_Issue_1_2015.pdf. Accessed June 16, 2016.

Gupta, A. (2010). Racial differences in response to antihypertensive therapy: Does one size fits all? *International Journal of Preventive Medicine,* Fall 2010, *1*(4), 217–219. PMCID: PMC3075515.

Hall, H., Li, J., & McKenna, M. (2005). HIV in predominantly rural areas of the United States. *The Journal of Rural Health,* Summer 2005, *21*(3), 245–253.

Health Resources and Services Administration (HRSA). (2010). *HRSA care action newsletter.* (Internet) http://hab.hrsa.gov/newspublications/careactionnewsletter/april2010.pdf

Heckman, T. G., Somlai, A. M., Peters, J., Walker, J., Otto-Salaj, L., Galdabini, C. A., et al. (1998). Barriers to care among persons living with HIV/AIDS in urban and rural areas. *AIDS Care, 10*(3), 365–375.

Hightow-Weidman, L., Muessig, K., Soni, K., Pike, E., Kirschke-Schwartz, H., & LeGrand, S. (2015, December). *Abstracts of the 2016 National HIV Prevention Conference.* Atlanta, GA. Abstract 2317.

HIV Specialist. (2016, March). *In crisis: The HIV workforce.* (Internet) http://onlinedigeditions. com/article/In+Crisis%3A+The+HIV+Workforce/2435156/0/article.html. Accessed June 16, 2016.

Hubach, R., Dodge, B., Li, M., Schick, V., Herbenick, D., Ramos W., … Reece, M. (2015). Loneliness, HIV-related stigma, and condom use among a predominantly rural sample of HIV-positive men who have sex with men (MSM). *AIDS Education and Prevention, 27*(1), 72–83.

Human Resource and Services Administration (HRSA). (2010, April). *HRSA care action.* (Internet) http://hab.hrsa.gov/newspublications/careactionnewsletter/april2010.pdf. Accessed June 16, 2016.

International Antiviral Society-USA. (2016). *Cases on the web.* https://www.iasusa.org/cow/

Lancaster Family Medicine Residency Curriculum. (2016). (Internet) http://www. lancasterfamilymed.org/Our-Program/Curriculum.aspx. Accessed June 17, 2016.

Langebeek, N., Gisolf, E. H., Reiss, P., Vervoort, S. C., Hafsteinsdóttir, T. B., Richter, C., … Nieuwkerk, P. T. (2014). Predictors and correlates of adherence to combination antiretroviral therapy (ART) for chronic HIV infection: A meta-analysis. *BMC Medicine, 12*(142), 140.

Medscape Public Health and Prevention. (2014). *Test your HIV patient care strategies.* http:// www.medscape.org/viewarticle/831237

O'Neill, M., Gregory, D., Karelas, G. D., Feller, D. J., Knudsen-Strong, E., Lajeunesse, D., … Agins, B. D. (2015). The HIV workforce in New York State: Does patient volume correlate with quality? *Clinical Infectious Diseases, 61*(12), 1871–1877, first published online September 30, 2015. doi:10.1093/cid/civ719

Padgett, P., Risser, J., Khuwaja, S., Lopez, Z., & Troisi, C. (2015, December). Homonegativity and depression among men who have sex with men. *Abstracts of the 2016 National HIV Prevention Conference.* Abstract 2210.

Ribaudo, H. J., Smith, K. Y., Robbins, G. K., Flexner, C., Haubrich, R., Chen, Y., et al. (2013). Racial differences in response to antiretroviral therapy for HIV infection: An AIDS Clinical Trials Group (ACTG) study analysis. *Clinical Infectious Diseases.* Presented in part: 18th conference on retroviruses and opportunistic infections, February 27–March 02, 2011. Abstract 50. doi:10.1093/cid/cit/595

Rosser, B., & Johnson, B. (2001, August). Evaluation of HIV prevention for men who have sex with men in thirteen rural states of the USA. *Abstracts of the 2001 National HIV Prevention Conference.* Atlanta, GA. Abstract 396.

Rural Health Information Hub, Georgia. (2015). https://www.ruralhealthinfo.org/states/georgia

Siddiqi, A., Hall, H. I., Hu, X., & Song, R. (2016). Population-based estimates of life expectancy after HIV diagnosis. United States 2008–2011. *JAIDS Journal of Acquired Immune Deficiency Syndromes* (publish ahead of print). doi:10.1097/QAI.0000000000000960

Sitron, J., Hawkins, L., Schlupp, A., Franklin, J., Johnson, C., & Brady, K. (2015, December). Understanding the social networks of young men who have sex with men: Formative ethnographic findings from the NHBS-YMSM pilot project. *Abstracts of the 2016 National HIV Prevention Conference.* Atlanta, GA. Abstract 2013.

Southern AIDS Manifesto Update. (2008). *A report of the Southern AIDS coalition.*

State Office of Rural Health, Georgia. (2015). http://dch.georgia.gov/sorh-maps-georgia-0. Accessed February 18, 2016.

The Los Angeles County HIV Public Health Fellowship. (2016). (Internet) http://www. lachivphfellowship.com/

Turan, B., Smith, W., Cohen, M., Wilson, T., Adimora, A., Merenstein D., … Turan, J. M. (2016). Mechanisms for the negative effects of internalized HIV-related stigma on ART adherence in women: The mediating roles of social isolation and depression. *JAIDS Journal of Acquired Immune Deficiency Syndromes* (publish ahead of print). doi:10.1097/QAI.0000000000000948

United States Department of Agriculture (USDA). (2013). *Rural-urban continuum codes.* http:// www.ers.usda.gov/data-products/rural-urban-continuum-codes/.aspx

Van Handel, M., Rose, C., Hallisey, E., Kolling, J., Zibbell, J., Lewis, B., … Brooks, J. (2016, June). County-level vulnerability assessment for rapid dissemination of HIV or HCV infections among persons who inject drugs, United States. *JAIDS Journal of Acquired Immune Deficiency Syndromes* (published ahead-of-print). doi:10.1097/QAI.0000000000001098

Visser, M. J., Kershaw, T., Matkin, J. D., & Forsyth, B. W. C. (2008). Development of parallel scales to measure HIV-related stigma. *AIDS Behavior, 12,* 759–771.

Vyavaharkar, M., Glover, S., Leonhirth, D., & Probst, J. (2013, January). *HIV/AIDS in Rural America: Prevalence and service availability.* South Carolina Rural Health Research Center. http://rhr.sph.sc.edu. Accessed February 18, 2016.

Williams, M., Bowen, A., & Horvath, K. (2005). The social/sexual environment of gay men residing in a rural frontier state: Implications for the development of HIV prevention programs. *The Journal of Rural Health, 21*(1), 48–55.

Chapter 2
More than Our Share: The Unchecked HIV/AIDS Crisis in Mississippi

Susan Hrostowski

Introduction

Rich and varied cultures as well as rich and varied geography make Mississippi a charming state. Mississippi has provided the world with talented musicians, gifted authors, and many creative individuals who have shaped American culture. There is beauty in the century-old oaks trees, power in the mighty Mississippi River, excitement in the sun and sand of the gulf coast, and grace in the abundance of fragrant azalea bushes. Underneath the veneer of southern gentility and beauty, however, there is a tangled and disparaging world of hardship and disparity. There are layers of dark history that have left deep gouges in the metaphorical landscape and continue to impact much of everyday life for the residents of the state. The horrors of slavery and segregation still echo throughout Mississippi, and prevailing conservative Christian values have profound effects on social welfare policy. Meanwhile, modern societal problems such as extreme poverty, racism, and substandard education tear at the fabric of Mississippi society. Mississippi's place as last in the country in almost every socioeconomic category causes and exacerbates a host of deeper issues, and chief among them is the HIV/AIDS crisis, one of Mississippi's deadliest and yet most ignored problems.

S. Hrostowski (✉)
Social Work, The University of Southern Mississippi, 118 College Drive #5114, Hattiesburg, MS 39406, USA
e-mail: susan.hrostowski@usm.edu

© Springer International Publishing AG 2017
F.M. Parks et al. (eds.), *HIV/AIDS in Rural Communities*,
DOI 10.1007/978-3-319-56239-1_2

Barriers to Curbing HIV in Mississippi

According to Reif, Geonnotti, and Whetten, (2006), factors that contribute to the spread of the HIV/AIDS epidemic in the South include stigma, conservativism, high rates of STIs, disparity, and poverty. Poor health literacy and poor education contribute to the stigma surrounding HIV and AIDS (Rosenberg, Broad, Mehlsak, Clark, & Greenwald, 2010). Many Mississippians including people with HIV do not know the facts about the disease, its causes, its modes of transmission, or its treatments. Stigma prevents people from getting tested and from getting treated, and results in discrimination against people who are infected with HIV. Research shows that

> Lack of knowledge about one's serostatus may in turn lead to inadvertent transmission of the virus and delays in the initiation of treatment. Second, among those who have been tested and are HIV-positive, stigma constitutes a chronic stressor that may contribute to coping difficulties, inadequate self-care, and difficulties with safer sex negotiation and condom use. (Venable, Carey, Blair, & Littlewood, 2006, p. 473).

Mississippi's political and social conservatism precludes helpful legislation. From the beginning of the AIDS crisis, Mississippi's government has been reluctant (and sometimes adamantly opposed) to providing education, prevention, services, or care. The political and social atmosphere in Mississippi has long reaching consequences with conservative views leading to resistance in creating or funding services for people with HIV/AIDS. Proposals to establish and maintain two HIV/STD clinics; to fund education, prevention, and treatment services; to remove the prescription drug and testing limits Medicaid has for HIV; and to match funds provided by the Ryan White Care Act all died in committees of the Mississippi Legislature (H.B. 326, 2013; H.B. 343, 2013; H.B. 1321, 2003; H.B. 169, 1998). Stigma around HIV/AIDS is perpetuated by laws that make it a crime to expose others to HIV/AIDS. In Mississippi, it is a federal offense to expose another person to HIV knowingly. This includes spitting and biting, which have been proven to not be exposure risks (Miss. Code Ann. § 97-27-14(1)).

The stigma of homosexuality in Mississippi is currently being exacerbated by the passage of Mississippi House Bill 1523, "Protecting Freedom of Conscience from Government Discrimination Act" which defines marriage as the union of one man and one woman and also classifies sex as only appropriate in the confines of that specific definition of marriage. It also stipulates that counselors may refuse to provide services to lesbian, gay, bisexual, and transgender clients (H.B. 1523, 2016). The bill was signed into law by the governor and was to go into effect on July 1, 2016, but was enjoined by the sixth district court. The governor has appealed this injunction, and that appeal is pending in the Fifth District Court of Appeals at this time. When accepting an award from an anti-LGBT rights group, he said that Christians will "stand in line to be crucified" for this law (Villarreal, 2016).

Public schools in Mississippi are required to teach abstinence-only or abstinence-plus sex education (H.B. 999). Both curricula teach that sex within the confines of marriage is the best way to prevent unplanned pregnancies and sexually transmitted diseases, but neither curriculum teaches safe sex practices such as condom usage. Not surprisingly, Mississippi ranked third in the country in the rate of teenage pregnancy in 2014, with the rate being 55% higher than the national average and more than 250% higher than the state with the lowest teen pregnancy rate, Massachusetts (The National Campaign to Prevent Teen and Unwanted Pregnancy, 2016). Sexually transmitted diseases also ravage Mississippi. Ranking twelfth for syphilis, third gonorrhea, and fifth for chlamydia demonstrates the critical need for improved sex education and removal of barriers for prevention in Mississippi. STDs not only predict HIV infection but actually promote it by lowering the immune system during active STD infection (CDC, 2016). Clearly, more comprehensive sex education is needed, considering these high rates and the fact that nationwide one in four new HIV infections are among young adults aged 13–24.

Racial disparity plays a significant role in Mississippi's HIV/AIDS crisis, and the high rates of new infections are most prominent among African Americans. Although African Americans make up only 37.6% of Mississippi's population (QuickFacts Mississippi, 2015), 78% of all new infections are among African Americans (MS Department of Health, 2015), nine times the rate of white individuals. African Americans are also ten times more likely to die than White HIV-positive individuals (MS Department of Health, 2010). The reasons for this racial discrepancy are the same seen in other areas of health disparity: poverty, lack of education, and poor general health. Additionally, the stigma surrounding sexual orientation and HIV status is stronger in the African American community, compounding the stigma and the barriers to care it presents noted above.

Chief among the challenges in combatting HIV is Mississippi's poverty. With 21.5% of adults and 35% of children living below the federal poverty line, Mississippi is the poorest state in the union (QuickFacts Mississippi, 2015). Poverty, of course, means a lack of basic resources and a lack of access to resources. The lack of transportation is a significant problem for people in poverty and makes access to health care and other resources extremely difficult.

Mississippi's Unique Challenges

HIV infection rates in Mississippi are among the highest in the country. According to the CDC, "The lifetime risk of HIV diagnosis is highest in the District of Columbia, followed by Maryland, Georgia, Florida, Louisiana, New York, Texas, New Jersey, Mississippi, South Carolina, North Carolina, Delaware, and Alabama" (HIV and AIDS in the United States by Geographic Distribution). It is important to remember that African Americans in Mississippi are disproportionately affected with more than eight times the rate of infection as Whites. The capital city of Jackson has the fourth highest rate of new infections in the country and the highest rate in the country among black men who have sex with men (CDC, 2014). Mississippi as a whole ranks second in the rate of new infections among 13–24 year olds. Compared to all the other states in the union, Mississippi has twice the national rate of death from HIV/AIDS (AIDSVu, 2016). Lack of testing due to stigma and lack of linkage to care both contribute to these high rates. According to Dr. Leandro Mena with the University of Mississippi Medical Center, half of all Mississippians diagnosed as HIV-positive are not receiving treatment (Fowler, 2016). In the more rural areas, people may not have access to care.

In this environment, people who test positive for HIV and the agencies who serve them scramble for resources. In a study of 218 HIV-positive persons utilizing a Ryan White clinic through a rural health association, the participants identified their most pressing needs as housing, financial assistance to meet basic needs, education about HIV medications, transportation, and assistance with medications other than their HIV medications (Hrostowski & Camp, 2015). Many need assistance in purchasing psychotropic medications and medications for such conditions as diabetes, high blood pressure, and heart disease; all of which affect their HIV treatment.

Safe and secure housing is vital to the health and well-being of anyone, and especially to those who are HIV-positive. Homelessness has been correlated with an increased risk of HIV, and homeless people with HIV/AIDS experience a worsening of symptoms three to six times the rate of individuals with HIV/AIDS with stable housing (National Health Care for the Homeless, 2008). This is likely due to reduced access to care, which leads to higher rates of morbidity, hospitalization, and mortality (Reid, Vittinghoff, & Kushel, 2008). Kathryn Garner, Executive Director of AIDS Services Coalition in Hattiesburg says, "Housing is treatment, and those who do not have it are at a much greater risk of dying. It's almost impossible to stay in care if you don't have a place to live" (Garner, personal communication, 2016).

One program that addresses housing needs is Housing Opportunities for People with AIDS (HOPWA). Funded through the U.S. Department of Housing and Urban Development, HOPWA provides case management, housing assistance, and other supportive services to low-income individuals living with HIV/AIDS. The problem here is the formulary used to allocate funds to the states. The formula used by HOPWA is based on the total number of HIV/AIDS cases in each state from the beginning of the outbreak of the virus, and those who have died are also included. Southern states would be allocated much more money if the HOPWA formula provided funds to the states based on the number of individuals actually living with HIV/AIDS (Hrostowski & Camp, 2015). Without this support, many people living with HIV are homeless or living in unstable situations.

HIV medications are provided to many patients through Ryan White funding. But again, the formulary short-shrifts Mississippians. In Fiscal Year 2013, the Deep South received an average of $3111 per AIDS case, while the national average excluding these states was $3843. This inequity has grown smaller over the last decade but the formula used for the disbursement of Ryan White funds is based on the total number of HIV infections instead of the number of new infections (Southern AIDS Coalition, 2012). Also, the formula does not take into account factors such as rural areas lacking medical providers or the cost of transportation for individuals living in rural areas to travel to medical providers in other areas (Hrostowski & Camp, 2015).

Because the majority of new infections are among people in poverty, the majority (51%) of payments for medical care for Mississippians with HIV/AIDS comes from Medicaid. Had Mississippi chosen to expand Medicaid under the Affordable Care Act, many more people living with HIV would have had access to care. In fact, 89% of Mississippians with HIV/AIDS whose services are paid through Ryan White funds would have become eligible for Medicaid. Mississippi, however, refused to expand Medicaid, as did many other southern states (H.B. 285, 2013; Center for Health Law and Policy, 2013). Again viewing Mississippi through the lens of the southeastern region of the United States, Medicaid enrollment of individuals with HIV/AIDS reveals a disparity. The national average of enrollment is 26%, but enrollment in the South is 23%. Getting Medicaid coverage in the South is more difficult than in other states due to more limiting eligibility criteria for adults with dependent children. Furthermore, even when people living with HIV or AIDS in the South have Medicaid, Medicaid will often limit the number of prescriptions covered, which can greatly affect a person who is already ill and living in poverty (Kaiser Family Foundation, 2011). Although the federal government pays Mississippi $3 for every $1 spent, Mississippi spends much less per individual than average for the nation. Specifically, the national average spent is a thousand dollars more per individual than what Mississippi spends, although Mississippi is receiving federal funds at the highest possible level (Human Rights Watch, 2011). Mississippi's income maximum for Medicaid eligibility is 46% of the federal poverty level, but the national cap is 66%.

As noted earlier, the lack of transportation is a problem for many Mississippians. Public transportation is only available in the larger cities, and even in those cities it is often limited. The SHARP report for Mississippi states

> In poor, rural areas, many residents do not have cars. Even if households have a vehicle, family members may have to share access to it, and may not be able to afford gas, maintenance, or insurance costs. Cars may be unreliable over long distances, such as highway travel; because of the rural nature of Mississippi, the nearest provider might be far away (Rosenberg et al., 2010, p. 57).

Advocates and Champions

In spite of the seemingly insurmountable problems and barriers to preventing HIV infection and helping people who are infected with or affected by HIV, Mississippi does have its HIV advocates and champions. In addition to the governmental agencies, such as the Department of Health, there are a few private, nonprofit AIDS service organizations (ASO's). As of this writing, there are four functioning ASO's in Mississippi. My Brother's Keeper (MBK) serves people in the Jackson metropolitan area and the Mississippi Gulf Coast, Grace House is also in Jackson,

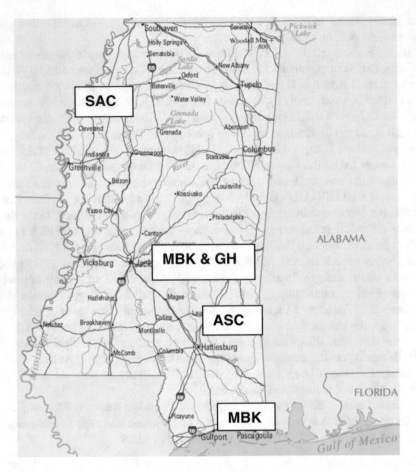

Fig. 2.1 MBK serves people in the Jackson metropolitan area and the Mississippi Gulf Coast

AIDS Services Coalition (ASC) is located in Hattiesburg and serves the mid-south region of the state, and the Southern AIDS Coalition (SAC) serves the Mississippi Delta. See Fig. 2.1. An ASO on the Mississippi Gulf Coast recently closed its doors due to financial difficulties. Telehealth services, in filling these service gaps, are a part of the Mississippi Department of Health's Statewide Comprehensive HIV Plan, but have yet to be implemented (MDH, 2012a, b).

The executive directors of these organizations spend a disproportionate amount of their time searching for funding to stay open and resources to serve their clients. Kathryn Garner of ASC states, "In other states, non-clinical agencies that provide supportive services to persons living with HIV share in Ryan White funding or in state-allocated funding. The Mississippi Legislature barely funds the required match each year, so funding for all but the medical and medication basics is but a wish"

(Garner, personal communication, 2016). In the last 2 years, two of the five ASO's in Mississippi have closed their doors. One of these agencies provided vital nutrition and supportive services in Jackson—where HIV rates for African American gay males by 2020 are expected to show that one in two are infected. The other was one of only three in Mississippi providing housing. Resources such as mental health care, treatment for addictions, transportation, housing, and employment opportunities are often limited and difficult to access.

> SHARP participants report a fragmented community structure and comment that cooperation and collaboration among ASOs, CBOs, and other providers is limited. This is probably due, at least in part, to competition for very limited resources. Compounding the issue is the fact that Mississippi has very few ASOs—some parts of the state, like northeast Mississippi, have no ASOs. There are very few "one-stop" ASOs that provide prevention education and testing, as well as supportive services like case management. There has also not been a consistent, statewide HIV/AIDS grassroots advocacy network, again probably at least partly due to a lack of resources (Rosenberg et al., 2010, p. 53).

Outlook

Unfortunately, resources are becoming even scarcer at this writing. Mississippi's state budget is in crisis. The State of Mississippi's 2017 budget has been drastically reduced from previous years due to revenue shortfalls and new tax cuts for businesses (Pender, 2016). Because of the cuts in state funding, Mississippi will lose even more in federal funds, because the state cannot meet the match requirement. Most departments will see sizeable funding cuts, leading to reductions in staff and services. The Department of Health is cutting at least 64 medical professionals from its staff and substantially reducing the services it renders to communities. In light of its 4.4% or $8.3 million-dollar budget cut, the Department of Mental Health will decrease the number of available psychiatric beds by more than 30 and the number of substance abuse treatment beds by about 67. There will no longer be a state-operated male chemical dependency unit in the state (Gates, 2016). These cuts along with the dismantling of the vocational rehabilitation services directly affect people with HIV/AIDS who rely on these departments for essential services.

Dr. Thomas Dobbs, the state epidemiologist, said in an interview that Mississippi's government has not considered the broader effects of its policies.

> Because we don't fund public health, we are a slave to federal programs and can't use the money we get from them in creative ways that meet the unique needs of Mississippians. The real tragedy in the systematic destruction of the public health system that can't respond to usual health concerns, let alone outbreaks of diseases. This makes it impossible to plan for the future (Dobbs, personal communication, 2016).

Dr. Dobbs went on to say that because of governmental antipathy, the local infrastructures are so limited that they cannot implement new interventions effectively, making responses to HIV less than optimal. Because Mississippi is not participating in the ACA, options for funding are limited. More outreach is needed to address the HIV epidemic, but the staff and the structures are not in place to carry it out.

Conclusion

The current situation and the foreseeable future are grim for Mississippians battling HIV, for people who are infected with or affected by HIV, for patients, families, friends, and service providers. Without fundamental changes in the values and mores, in the culture, of the people of Mississippi, changes in the state's approach to HIV will not occur. Homophobia, racism, and ignorance exacerbate the crisis. Policies created by legislators with these mindsets restrict the dissemination of prevention and treatment information, discourage people from getting tested, and inhibit the delivery of services.

References

AIDSVu. (2016). *Age-adjusted rates of death due to HIV disease, 2011–2013*. Retrieved from http://aidsvu.org/state/mississippi/

An Act to Amend Section 37-13-171, Mississippi Code Of 1972, To Require Each Local School Board to Adopt a Sex-Related Education Policy to Implement Abstinence-Only or Abstinence-Plus Education into Its Local School District's Curriculum by June 30, 2012, or to Require the Local School Board to Adopt the Program Developed by the Mississippi Department of Human Services and the Department of Health; To Require The State Department to Approve Each District's Curriculum for Sex-Related Education and Establish a Protocol to Be Used by Districts to Provide Continuity in Teaching the Approved Curriculum; To Provide That Instruction in School Districts Implementing Abstinence-Plus Education into the Curriculum May Be Expanded Beyond the Instruction for Abstinence-Only Education within Parameters Approved by the Department; To Define Abstinence-Plus Education; To Remove the Authority Given to Local School Boards to Vote in Favor of Teaching Sex Education without any Instruction on Abstinence; To Prohibit any Teaching that Abortion Can Be Used to Prevent the Birth of a Baby; To Require Boys and Girls to Be Separated into Different Classes by Gender at All Times When Sex-Related Education Is Discussed or Taught; To Require the Department of Human Services and the Department of Health to Develop Certain Programs and Strategies Promoting Pregnancy Prevention and Providing Information on the Consequences of Unprotected, Uninformed and Underage Sexual Activity; To Provide for the Repeal of this Section on July 1, 2016; To Amend Section 37-13-173, Mississippi Code of 1972, Relating to Parental Notice; To Amend Section 2 Chapter 507, Laws of 2009, To Revise the Duties of the Teen Pregnancy Prevention Task Force and to Extend the Date of the Repeal on the Task Force to July 1, 2016; to Require the State Department of Health and the State Department Of Education, Subject to the Availability of Funds, To Establish a Pilot Program in Each Health Care District, To Be Located in a School District in a County Having the Highest Number of Teen Pregnancies; To Require those Agencies to Provide Certain Educational Services through Qualified Personnel; and for Related Purposes, MS H.B. 999, Regular Session (2011).

An Act to Amend Section 43-13-115, Mississippi code of 1972, to Provide Medicaid Coverage for Individuals who are Under 65 Years of Age, are not pregnant, are not Entitled to or Enrolled for Medicare Benefits and Whose Income is not More Than 133% of the Federal Poverty Level, as Authorized Under the Federal Patient Protection and Affordable Care Act; to Provide Medicaid Coverage for Children who are Under 19 Years of Age and Whose Family Income is More Than 133% but not More Than 200% of the Federal Poverty Level, as Authorized Under the Children's Health Insurance Program; to Repeal Section 41-86-1, 41-86-5, 41-86-7, 41-86-9, 41-86-11, 41-86-13 and 41-86-15, Mississippi Code of 1972, Which are the Mississippi Children's Health Insurance Program Act; and for Related Purposes, MS H.B. 285, Regular Session (2013).

An Act to Amend Section 43-13-117, Mississippi Code of 1972, To Prohibit the Division of Medicaid from Establishing Limits or Restrictions on Drugs or Tests Prescribed for the Treatment and Prevention of HIV/AIDS or Hepatitis C; and For Related Purposes, MS H.B. 1321, Regular Session (2003).

An Act To Create The "Protecting Freedom Of Conscience From Government Discrimination Act"; To Provide Certain Protections Regarding A Sincerely Held Religious Belief Or Moral Conviction For Persons, Religious Organizations And Private Associations; To Define A Discriminatory Action For Purposes Of This Act; To Provide That A Person May Assert A Violation Of This Act As A Claim Against The Government; To Provide Certain Remedies; To Require A Person Bringing A Claim Under This Act To Do So Not Later Than Two Years After The Discriminatory Action Was Taken; To Provide Certain Definitions; And For Related Purposes, H.B. 1523, Regular Session (2016).

An Act Making An Appropriation to the State Department of Health for the Purpose of Developing, Establishing, and Operating Two STD/HIV Specialty Clinics for the Fiscal Year 2014, MS H.B. 343, Regular Session (2013).

An Act Making an Appropriation to the State Department of Health for the Purpose of Providing Funds for HIV/AIDS Education, Prevention and Treatment Programs and Services for the Fiscal Year 2014, MS H.B. 326, Regular Session (2013).

An Act to Provide that the Legislature Shall Appropriate to the State Department of Health Annually from the State General Fund an Amount Equal to the Amount of the Grant that the State Receives from the Federal Government Under the Ryan White Care Grant Program; to Provide that these Funds Shall be a Separate Line Item in the Appropriation Bill of the Department; and Shall be Designated as Mississippi Ryan White Supplemental Funds; to Provide that the Department Shall Expend these Supplemental Funds Exclusively for HIV Disease Medications; and for Related Purposes, MS H.B. 169, Regular Session (1998).

Center for Disease Control and Prevention. (2014). *Sexually transmitted disease surveillance.* Retrieved from http://www.cdc.gov/hiv/statistics/index.html

Center for Disease Control and Prevention. (2016). *STDs and HIV—CDC Fact Sheet.* Retrieved from https://www.cdc.gov/std/hiv/stdfact-std-hiv.htm

Center for Health Law and Policy Innovation of Harvard Law School and the Treatment Access Expansion Project. (2013). *State Health Reform Impact Model Project: Mississippi.* Retrieved from http://www.hivhealthreform.org/wp-content/uploads/2013/03/Mississippi-Modeling-Report-Final.pdf

Contagious diseases; causing exposure to human immunodeficiency virus (HIV), hepatitis B or hepatitis C; crime of endangerment by bodily substance; violations and penalties. § 97-27-14.

Dobbs, T. (2016, July 11). Personal interview.

Fowler, S. (2016, May). HIV rate among Jackson gay, bisexual men highest in US. *The Clarion Ledger.* Retrieved from http://www.clarionledger.com/story/news/2016/05/17/gay-men-hiv-southern-cities/84523790/

Garner, K. (2016, June 5). Personal interview.

Gates, J. (2016). Mississippi budget cuts to close psychiatric beds. *The Clarion-Ledger.* Retrieved from http://www.clarionledger.com/story/news/2016/05/10/state-budget-cuts-close-psychiatric-beds/84181292/

Human Rights Watch. (2011). *Rights at risk: State response to HIV in Mississippi*. Retrieved from http://www.hrw.org/sites/default/files/reports/us0311web_0.pdf

Hrostowski, S., & Camp, A. (2015). The unchecked HIV/AIDS crisis in Mississippi. *Social Work in Health Care, 54*(5), 474–483. doi:10.1080/00981389.2015.1030057.

Kaiser Family Foundation. (2011 & 2011a). Retrieved from http://kff.org/hivaids/fact-sheet/the-hivaids-epidemic-in-the-united-states/

Mississippi State Department of Health. (2010). *State of Mississippi 2010 STD/HIV epidemiologic profile*. Retrieved from http://www.healthyms.com/msdhsite/_static/resources/3591.pdf

Mississippi State Department of Health. (2012a). *HIV care and treatment program*. Retrieved from http://msdh.ms.gov/msdhsite/_static/14,13047,150.html

Mississippi State Department of Health. (2012b). *2012 Statewide comprehensive HIV plan and statewide coordinated statement of need*. Retrieved from http://msdh.ms.gov/msdhsite/_static/resources/5714.pdf

Mississippi QuickFacts. (2015). *United States Census Bureau*. Retrieved from https://www.census.gov/quickfacts/table/PST045215/28

National Health Care for the Homeless Council. (2008). *Health care for the homeless: Comprehensive services to meet complex needs*. Retrieved from http://www.nhchc.org/wp-content/uploads/2011/10/HCHbrochure2008.pdf

Pender, G. (2016). State agencies pondering cuts, layoffs with new budget. *The Clarion-Ledger*. Retrieved from http://www.clarionledger.com/story/news/politics/2016/05/01/state-budget-cuts/83699348/

Reid, K. W., Vittinghoff, E., & Kushel, M. B. (2008). Association between the level of housing instability, economic standing and health care access: A meta-regression. *Journal of Health Care for the Poor and Underserved, 19*(4), 1212–1228. doi:10.1353/hpu.0.0068.

Reif, S., Geonnotti, K. L., & Whetten, K. (2006). HIV infection and AIDS in the deep south. *American Journal of Public Health, 96*(6), 970–973.

Rosenberg, A., Broad, E., Mehlsak, R., Clark, S., & Greenwald, R. (2010). *Mississippi State Report: An analysis of the successes, challenges, and opportunities for improving healthcare access*. Retrieved from http://www.taepusa.org/Portals/0/Documents/Mississippi%20SHARP%20report.pdf

Southern AIDS Coalition. (2012). *Southern AIDS Manifesto: Update 2012*. Retrieved from http://southernaidscoalition.org/wp-content/uploads/2013/11/Southern-States-Manifesto-Update-2012.pdf

Venable, P. A., Carey, M. P., Blair, D. C., & Littlewood, R. A. (2006). Impact of HIV-related stigma on health behaviors and psychological adjustment among HIV-positive men and women. *AIDS and Behavior, 10*, 473–482.

Villarreal, Y. (2016). Mississippi Gov.: Christians willing to be crucified to protect anti-LGBT law. *Advocate*. Retrieved from http://www.advocate.com/politics/2016/6/01/mississippi-gov-christians-willing-be-crucified-protect-anti-lgbt-law

Part II
HIV Disease and Primary Care

Chapter 3
HIV/AIDS: The Last 30-Plus Years

Anne Marie Schipani-McLaughlin, Danielle Lambert,
Carolyn Lauckner and Nathan Hansen

Origin and Early History of HIV/AIDS

The HIV/AIDS epidemic was first recognized in the United States in 1981 when a small subset of gay men in California started showing unusual physical symptoms that drew the attention of doctors, public health officials, and the media (U.S. Department of Health and Human Services, 2015). On June 5, 1981, the Centers for Disease Control and Prevention (CDC) released its first Morbidity and Mortality Weekly Report (MMWR) on what they thought were cases of a rare lung infection called Pneumocystis carinii pneumonia (PCP) in five gay and previously healthy men in Los Angeles, California. All men had weakened immune systems and

A.M. Schipani-McLaughlin (✉) · D. Lambert
Department of Health Promotion and Behavior, University of Georgia
College of Public Health, 242 Wright Hall, 100 Foster Rd,
Health Sciences Campus, Athens, GA 30602, USA
e-mail: Annemarie.schipani25@uga.edu

D. Lambert
e-mail: dnl@uga.edu

C. Lauckner
Department of Health Promotion and Behavior, University of Georgia
College of Public Health, 321B Wright Hall, 100 Foster Rd,
Health Sciences Campus, Athens, GA 30602, USA
e-mail: clauck@uga.edu

N. Hansen
Department of Health Promotion and Behavior, University of Georgia
College of Public Health, 131 Wright Hall, 100 Foster Rd,
Health Sciences Campus, Athens, GA 30602, USA
e-mail: nhansen@uga.edu

© Springer International Publishing AG 2017
F.M. Parks et al. (eds.), *HIV/AIDS in Rural Communities*,
DOI 10.1007/978-3-319-56239-1_3

showed other symptoms aside from PCP. From the onset of their symptoms to the time the report was released, two out of the five infected men had already died. This report marks CDC's first official reporting on the AIDS epidemic (CDC, 1981). With this report began a flood of attention from the media and doctors around the country reporting similar symptoms in patients. Soon after the MMWR release on PCP in 1981 and other reported cases of opportunistic infections, CDC also reported 26 cases of Kaposi's sarcoma, a rare cancer, among young gay men in Los Angeles, New York City, and San Francisco (Haverkos & Curran, 1982; U.S. Department of Health and Human Services, 2015). At the forefront of the epidemic, scientists rapidly tried to understand the disease to prevent its continuous spread.

Early research on the HIV/AIDS epidemic strove to understand the etiology, causes, and routes of transmission, and track the epidemiology and disease spread. In 1982, the CDC used the term *acquired immune deficiency syndrome*, or AIDS, for the first time with the following case definition: "a disease at least moderately predictive of a defect in cell-mediated immunity, occurring in a person with no known case for diminished resistance to that disease" (U.S. Department of Health and Human Services, 2015). As the disease continued to spread, the government designated millions of dollars in funding to CDC and National Institutes of Health (NIH) to increase disease surveillance and scientific research. With this, scientific understanding of the disease increased.

In September 1983, the CDC released an MMWR identifying the groups most affected by AIDS and ruled out disease transmission via casual contact, food, water, air, and environmental surfaces. Though the disease was mainly thought to affect gay men up until this point, the CDC saw its first AIDS case contracted through a blood transfusion and the first AIDS cases in women in which AIDS was transmitted through sexual contact (U.S. Department of Health and Human Services, 2015). The CDC noted that the main populations affected by AIDS included men identifying as gay or bisexual, intravenous drug users, and hemophiliacs (Centers for Disease Control and Prevention, 1983). Despite the scientific advancements and furthered understanding of HIV, the disease continued to spread and, by 1985, at least one AIDS case had been reported in every region of the world (U.S. Department of Health and Human Services, 2015).

In the same MMWR, the CDC noted that most cases reported to surveillance occurred among residents in large urban U.S. cities (Centers for Disease Control and Prevention, 1983). At the beginning of the HIV/AIDS epidemic in the United States, urban cities were considered the epicenter of the epidemic despite the fact that rural America suffered as well (Driesbach, 2009). This brings into question whether HIV/AIDS cases in rural areas were unrecognized, unreported, or ignored during the early epidemic, and how this may have reflected and affected the level of HIV/AIDS-related knowledge in rural communities at the forefront of the epidemic (Centers for Disease Control and Prevention, 1983; Driesbach, 2009).

Stigma and Discrimination

From the very start of the epidemic, men who have sex with men (MSM) faced discrimination and stigma related to HIV/AIDS, which was labeled by many as a "gay man's disease." Even doctors faced stigma and discrimination for treating patients with HIV/AIDS; one New York City doctor, for example, was threatened with eviction from his building for treating AIDS patients. In 1985, Ryan White, a high school student who contracted AIDS through a blood transfusion when treated for hemophilia, spoke out publicly in the media against AIDS discrimination and stigma. Up until this point, U.S. President Ronald Reagan had not addressed the HIV/AIDS epidemic since it first surfaced in 1981. Soon after, Ryan White became a national figure advocating against HIV/AIDS and President Reagan publicly mentioned AIDS for the first time (U.S. Department of Health and Human Services, 2015). Despite these efforts, stigma and discrimination continued to affect persons living with HIV/AIDS (PLWHA), with many myths and misconceptions about how it is transmitted continuing to persist in the modern world. HIV/AIDS-related stigma has especially led to challenges addressing the epidemic within rural communities in the United States. Rural communities face inherent challenges such as lack of education, limited job opportunities, and inadequate access to health care and social services. Added social stigmas related to HIV/AIDS make HIV prevention and treatment particularly difficult in rural communities (Driesbach, 2009).

The early religious response to HIV/AIDS also contributed to stigma and prevention efforts. For example, the Catholic Church's religious views on homosexuality and birth control shaped their initial view on HIV/AIDS, with their response suggesting that individuals should not rely on condoms to prevent HIV/AIDS and that condoms could make the problem worse by encouraging more sexual behavior (Benagiano, Carrara, Filippi, & Brosens, 2011). Within religious organizations a lack of HIV/AIDS-related education, negative messages about how the virus is spread and those living with the virus, and misinformation about methods of prevention may contribute to misconceptions and stigma related to HIV/AIDS. Because evidence suggests that those living in rural communities or primarily rural areas in the United States have higher levels of religiosity than those in urban areas (Dillon & Savage, 2006; Lipka & Wormald, 2016), such beliefs can have an especially significant effect on rural HIV/AIDS stigma, prevention, and treatment. While there has been a positive shift with some Christian churches providing HIV education and testing, particularly among Black/African American communities (Berkley-Patton et al., 2010; McNeal & Perkins, 2007), religion is likely to remain an important factor to consider when addressing HIV/AIDS in rural areas.

Policy and Advocacy Responses to HIV/AIDS

Early response to the epidemic took place on global, national, and local levels. In 1985, the World Health Organization (WHO) and the U.S. Department of Health and Human Services held the first International AIDS Conference in Atlanta, Georgia. In 1988, in recognition of the fact that HIV/AIDS affected individuals around the globe, the WHO declared December 1 as World AIDS Day. On a national level, early response efforts involved legislature, advocacy, and government funding to support HIV/AIDS research. The first congressional hearing on HIV/AIDS was held in 1982, where the CDC estimated that AIDS would affect thousands of people. That same year, legislation designated funding to CDC and NIH to support HIV/AIDS research. President Reagan drew further attention to the epidemic when he wrote a letter to Congress in order to make HIV/AIDS a priority in 1985. After Ryan White died of AIDS-related illnesses in 1990, the U.S. Congress enacted the Ryan White Comprehensive AIDS Resource Emergency (CARE) Act of 1990, which designated millions of dollars in federal funding for HIV/AIDS community-based care and treatment efforts (U.S. Department of Health and Human Services, 2015). Local HIV/AIDS prevention in the United States occurred through grassroots community mobilization, particularly in urban cities such as San Francisco and New York City. Many urban U.S. cities, including San Francisco, New York City, and Los Angeles, closed bathhouses due to high-risk sexual activity that occurred within and contributed to the spread of the epidemic. However, rural U.S. communities were absent from the national conversation on HIV/AIDS at the beginning of the epidemic (Driesbach, 2009).

Many policy decisions made during this time had an effect on the way that society as a whole viewed HIV/AIDS. For example, in 1987, the U.S. Public Health Service added HIV as a "contagious infectious disease" to the immigrant exclusion list and enforced all HIV testing for all U.S. visa applicants. This policy change had a ripple effect on the United States, affecting future policy changes and stigma attached to HIV/AIDS. In 1990, the sixth International AIDS Conference was held in San Francisco but domestic and international nonprofit organizations boycotted the conference to protest the U.S. immigration policy banning those with HIV from entering the country. The eighth International AIDS Conference in 1992 was set to be held in Boston, but was moved to Amsterdam again due to the U.S. immigration restrictions on people living with HIV/AIDS. In 2009, President Obama announced that his administration would officially lift the HIV travel and immigration ban in January 2010 and remove the final barriers to entry. Lifting the travel ban occurred alongside the announcement that the 2012 International AIDS Conference would be held in Washington, DC, the first time in over 20 years that the conference was held in the United States (U.S. Department of Health and Human Services, 2015). Efforts such as these by President Obama are critical in addressing the problem of stigma and discrimination related to PLWHA.

Many community-based advocacy organizations have also sought to reduce HIV/AIDS discrimination, increase education and awareness, and aid those living with HIV/AIDS. In 1984, several AIDS service organizations banded together to form AIDS Action, a national organization based out of Washington, DC, that advocated on behalf of individuals and communities affected by HIV/AIDS, provided HIV/AIDS-related education to the Federal government, and helped shape HIV/AIDS-related policies and regulations (U.S. Department of Health and Human Services, 2015). Other grassroots AIDS advocacy organizations were developed to serve special populations affected by the epidemic, such as MSM, individuals with hemophilia, African Americans, women, and children (U.S. Department of Health and Human Services, 2015). For example, in 1988, Elizabeth Glaser, an HIV-positive mother with two HIV-positive children, formed an organization with two friends, the Elizabeth Glaser Pediatric AIDS Foundation, which advocated for research on HIV treatment and care for children living with HIV/AIDS (U.S. Department of Health and Human Services, 2015). Faith-based nonprofit organizations, such as the National AIDS Interfaith Network, have also played an important role in HIV/AIDS advocacy, education, and care. The National AIDS Interfaith Network was founded in 1986 to educate the faith community on HIV/AIDS and link individuals living with HIV and AIDS to appropriate services (U.S. Department of Health and Human Services, 2015).

Early in the epidemic, most of these advocacy organizations were based out of major urban cities such as Los Angeles, New York, San Francisco, and Washington, DC, though today there are thousands of HIV/AIDS organizations throughout the country located in urban and rural areas alike (Driesbach, 2009; U.S. Department of Health and Human Services, 2015). However, rural community organizations achieved success using different strategies than urban advocacy groups (Driesbach, 2009; Rural Center for AIDS/STD Prevention, 2009; Topping & Hartwig, 1997). The traditional San Francisco, CA model for delivering HIV services to the community, which served as the basis for the Robert Wood Johnson Foundation AIDS Health Service Program, does not work as well in rural communities because it focuses heavily on advocacy and, in rural communities, advocacy can conflict with provision of services. Instead, rural communities have had success in HIV prevention, education, and treatment by sharing resources within the community between nonprofit organizations, schools, health departments, and healthcare providers (Driesbach, 2009; Rural Center for AIDS/STD Prevention, 2009; Topping & Hartwig, 1997). These rural organizations have made significant strides in addressing HIV/AIDS among these communities, but much work remains to be done.

Populations Affected by HIV/AIDS in the Past 30 Years

With the first MMWR in June 1981, the epidemic has largely been associated with MSM (Centers for Disease Control and Prevention, 2006a; De Cock, Jaffe, & Curran, 2011). This initial publication specifically tied the illness to "homosexual men" and suggested the spread was directly related to gender-specific sexual behaviors, commencing the HIV-related stigmatization and misconceptions still common today (De Cock et al., 2011; Goldin, 1994; Parker & Aggleton, 2003; Preston et al., 2004). Other risk groups identified early in the outbreak included injection drug users and transfusion recipients, leading researchers to recognize primary modes of transmission as sexual contact and blood. The appearance of the virus in infants and young children also led to the discovery of mother-to-child transmission (Cummins et al., 2016; De Cock et al., 2011). While MSM remain most affected by new diagnoses of HIV, a myriad of other populations are now acknowledged as being disproportionately affected by the epidemic, particularly ethnic and racial minorities (Centers for Disease Control and Prevention, 2006a). African American and Hispanic communities represent a small proportion of the larger U.S. population, but have significantly higher rates of infection compared to Whites. Women have also emerged as a high-risk population, now second to MSM for new HIV infections, with transmission from heterosexual contact continuing to rise (Centers for Disease Control and Prevention, 2006a, 2015b).

As mentioned, the HIV epidemic has historically focused on prevalence, prevention, and treatment in large metropolitan or urban areas of the United States (Berry, 1993). Although urban areas saw the greatest increase in HIV cases from 1982 to 1984, the 25 counties with the greatest increase in HIV cases from 1988 to 1990 were rural areas (Lam & Liu, 1994). The rise of HIV in rural America came with numerous challenges, many of which are still problematic today (Graham, Forrester, Wysong, Rosenthal, & James, 1995; Heckman, Somlai, Kelly, Stevenson, & Galdabini, 1996; Heckman et al., 1998; Smith, Landau, & Bahr, 2009; Sowell et al., 1997). Health professionals in rural areas had little experience diagnosing and treating individuals living with HIV; and health clinics and services were limited and often a considerable distance for individuals to travel, which was further complicated by the lack of transportation (Smith et al., 2009). Small close-knit communities made it difficult for individuals to seek care and resources confidentially, especially in rural areas where conservative moral values may perpetuate stigmatization and influence community norms (Dreisbach, 2009; Smith et al., 2009). Due to these challenges, individuals residing in rural areas have been shown to receive care from less experienced providers, are less likely to be prescribed antiretroviral medications, and experience greater stigmatization (Cohn et al., 2001; Graham et al., 1995; Sowell et al., 1997).

Considering the current disparities among racial minorities, MSM, women, and due to socio-contextual determinants of health, such as poverty and geographic location, HIV prevalence in the southeastern United States has become especially problematic (AIDSVu). Individuals living with HIV are highly concentrated in the Deep South, particularly in rural areas, as shown in Fig. 3.1, which also coincides with the greatest prevalence of African American communities, Hispanic communities, income inequality, male-to-male transmission, and heterosexual transmission (AIDSVu).

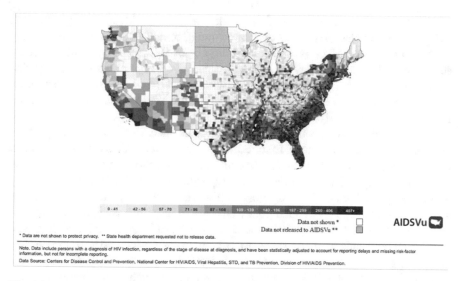

Fig. 3.1 Rates of persons living with an HIV diagnosis, by county, 2012. Photo courtesy of AIDSVu (aidsvu.org). Emory University, Rollins School of Public Health

Evolution of HIV Testing and Treatment

A key component of addressing HIV/AIDS and reducing its spread, in addition to policy and advocacy, is advancing research and science that can help to prevent, detect, and treat the disease. Testing and treatment for HIV/AIDS has evolved over time with more understanding of HIV/AIDS. In 1985, the Food and Drug Administration (FDA) first tested the blood supply in blood banks in order to detect HIV antibodies after individuals contracted the virus via blood transfusions. The FDA released the first commercial HIV test called ELISA in 1985 and, in 1987, the Western blood blot test kit was introduced as a specific test for HIV antibodies (U.S. Department of Health and Human Services, 2015). In 1987, the FDA released the first treatment for HIV, azidothymidine, or AZT. Later, the emergence of antiretroviral therapy, or ART, gave rise to the HIV treatment used currently, highly active antiretroviral therapy (HAART) (U.S. Department of Health and Human Services, 2015).

Advances in HIV testing technology over the last 30 years have assisted in addressing previously mentioned barriers to HIV prevention and linkage to care. Rapid testing, such as the OraQuick and INSTI tests, has made it possible to provide quick and accurate results in as little as one minute, increasing the number of individuals tested within a given time frame and allowing for immediate referral to treatment. Testing initiatives have now been mobilized in a variety of different settings due to the capabilities of rapid testing, as the previous need for laboratory access and multiple visits is eliminated. This aids in reducing barriers to clinic access and transportation, especially in rural areas. Rapid HIV testing also led to the availability of home test kits, which provide greater confidentiality by allowing individuals to purchase HIV tests over the counter, or online, and test in the privacy of their own home. This is particularly important in small communities where access to health services may be limited by perceived stigma and discomfort discussing personal sexual health behaviors with a local provider over privacy concerns (Centers for Disease Control and Prevention, 2016; The Henry J. Kaiser Family Foundation, 2016).

Currently, the CDC recommends all individuals aged 13–64 years be tested for HIV at least once as a part of routine health care. If individuals are engaging in high-risk behaviors, such as unsafe sex or sharing injection drug equipment, it is recommended that they get tested annually, with more frequent testing of every 3–6 months if individuals are engaging in high-risk behaviors with sexually active gay or bisexual men. HIV-related policy changes to insurance coverage through the Affordable Care Act in April 2013 increased the feasibility of routine testing, and revised recommendations for states to adhere to an opt-out HIV testing policy promoted greater uptake as well. Although HIV testing is typically voluntary, the United States mandates HIV testing for specific cases, such as for blood or organ donation, certain incarcerated individuals, individuals seeking to enter the military or active duty personnel, and, in some states, newborns (Centers for Disease Control and Prevention, 2016; The Henry J. Kaiser Family Foundation, 2016).

Research-Based Solutions to Address the HIV Epidemic

HIV prevention programs have evolved from grassroots efforts in 1982 among MSM in San Francisco and New York to public and private funding for a wide array of HIV-related research priorities. As research priorities have changed, programming has shifted from a focus on assessing disease prevalence and prevention through reducing risk behaviors (unprotected sex, injection drug use) to the current priorities of addressing the HIV care continuum and medical treatment as prevention. For consistent assessment of rigor, the CDC now evaluates the scientific evidence of HIV prevention and sexual risk reduction interventions. Those with good scientific support are designated evidence-based interventions (EBIs), the current standard for best practices in public health research and practice. These EBIs are packaged and available for community-based implementation to increase dissemination and sustainability efforts. PLWHA were excluded from early prevention programs and research, and it was not until 2001 when the CDC introduced a framework for addressing prevention and wellness among HIV-positive individuals that a change in research priorities began to occur (Centers for Disease Control and Prevention, 2006b).

Although research programs and interventions have successfully contributed to the understanding and prevention of HIV/AIDS, there is still a significant need to address challenges in order to reduce the growing number of HIV-related disparities. The vast majority of current research still focuses on urban areas, failing to recognize the needs of rural populations. Social inequalities and stigma, especially in rural communities, must be addressed alongside health services in order to reduce barriers to adequate and equal care. More research is also needed specifically for highly affected populations, such as sexual and racial minorities. Engaging health departments, clinics, and community partners in these research and prevention efforts is critical to improving the capacity and feasibility of all providers to translate research into an applied setting (Centers for Disease Control and Prevention, 2006b).

Lessons Learned and Future Directions

Throughout the previous 30 years, researchers, medical professionals, and advocates have learned a great deal about best practices for addressing and reducing the burden of HIV/AIDS. Policy and advocacy efforts have demonstrated their potential to shift community conversations about HIV, reduce stigma and discrimination, control the spread of the disease, and improve access to testing and treatment. Research has helped to determine effective methods of addressing HIV/AIDS at all points in the care continuum—from prevention, to diagnosis of HIV, to linkage to and retention in care, to prescription of ART, and to viral suppression. The development of EBIs, such as the Antiretroviral Treatment Access Study (ARTAS) that promotes retention in HIV care, or the AMIGAS intervention for reducing HIV risk among Latinas, have been especially beneficial, for improving the rigor of inquiry and encouraging the use of scientific approaches in addressing HIV/AIDS (Centers for Disease Control and Prevention, 2015a). However, the majority of these interventions are dedicated to prevention and risk reduction, while less work has been devoted to improved linkage to and retention in care, as well as medication adherence. Additionally, very few interventions have been targeted specifically toward rural populations, who face their own unique challenges related to HIV/AIDS.

The NIH has updated their research priorities to reflect these gaps in research, and is now focused on supporting research related to HIV treatment, vaccines, and the reduction in health disparities (National Institutes of Health, 2015). This increased emphasis on promoting linkage to care and reducing disparities will likely have important effects on rural populations at risk of or living with HIV, though there will still be a need to address issues of stigma and discrimination in these communities. Research to date has struggled to find rigorous and effective stigma-reduction interventions (Sengupta, Banks, Jonas, Miles, & Smith, 2011), so this will remain an important area of inquiry moving forward in terms of addressing rural HIV. Additionally, there are several other barriers associated with rural HIV care that demand attention, including a lack of a stable healthcare infrastructure, HIV workforce availability and turnover issues, and patients' ability to get transportation to health clinics (Health Resources and Services Administration, 2010; Reif, Golin, & Smith, 2005). These barriers are not easily addressed, but could potentially be managed through innovative applications of technology that can improve access, such as using videoconferencing to connect patients with HIV providers (Caceres, Gomez, Garcia, Gatell, & del Pozo, 2006). Such efforts, combined with advocacy and education, are needed to address the growing problem of HIV/AIDS in rural areas.

Conclusion

This review of the previous 30-plus years of the HIV/AIDS epidemic has sought to not only illustrate the significant strides that have been made in terms of reducing the spread of the disease and addressing issues of stigma and discrimination, but to also illustrate the steps that remain to be taken. Much of what we know about HIV/AIDS is the result of work that has been done in urban communities and with MSM. While these are important populations to address because of the high prevalence of HIV/AIDS, the impact of the disease on those living in rural areas has not been widely discussed or studied. The little research that has been done, however, has indicated that stigma toward HIV is common in rural communities and that those living with HIV/AIDS in such areas lack access to appropriate care (Smith et al., 2009; Sowell et al., 1997). Thus, despite the advances in treatment and testing that have helped to control the spread and effects of HIV, there are many challenges that need to be addressed. As we look ahead to the next 30 years of HIV/AIDS advocacy, services, and research, it is essential that we devote resources and attention to addressing the disease in rural areas.

References

AIDSVu. Emory University, Rollins School of Public Health. Retrieved from http://aidsvu.org/

Benagiano, G., Carrara, S., Filippi, V., & Brosens, I. (2011). Condoms, HIV and the roman catholic church. *Reproductive Biomedicine Online, 22*(7), 701–709.

Berkley-Patton, J., Bowe-Thompson, C., Bradley-Ewing, A., Hawes, S., Moore, E., Williams, E., … Goggin, K. (2010). Taking it to the pews: A CBPR-guided HIV awareness and screening project with black churches. *AIDS Education and Prevention: Official Publication of the International Society for AIDS Education, 22*(3), 218.

Berry, D. E. (1993). The emerging epidemiology of rural AIDS. *The Journal of Rural Health, 9*(4), 293–304.

Caceres, C., Gomez, E. J., Garcia, F., Gatell, J. M., & del Pozo, F. (2006). An integral care telemedicine system for HIV/AIDS patients. *International Journal of Medical Informatics, 75*(9), 638–642.

Centers for Disease Control and Prevention. (1981). *Pneumocystis pneumonia—Los Angeles.* Retrieved from Atlanta, GA: http://www.cdc.gov/mmwr/preview/mmwrhtml/june_5.htm

Centers for Disease Control and Prevention. (1983). *Current trends update: Acquired immunodeficiency syndrome (AIDS)—United States.* Retrieved from Atlanta, GA: http://www.cdc.gov/mmwr/preview/mmwrhtml/00000137.htm

Centers for Disease Control and Prevention. (2006a). Epidemiology of HIV/AIDS—United States, 1981–2005. *MMWR, 55*(21), 589–592.

Centers for Disease Control and Prevention. (2006b). Evolution of HIV/AIDS prevention programs—United States, 1981–2006. *MMWR, 55*(21), 597–603.

Centers for Disease Control and Prevention. (2015a). Compendium of evidence-based interventions and best practices for HIV prevention. Retrieved from http://www.cdc.gov/hiv/research/interventionresearch/compendium/index.html

Centers for Disease Control and Prevention. (2015b). HIV in the United States: At a glance. Retrieved from http://www.cdc.gov/hiv/statistics/overview/ataglance.html

Centers for Disease Control and Prevention. (2016). HIV/AIDS testing. Retrieved from http://www.cdc.gov/hiv/basics/testing.html

Cohn, S. E., Berk, M. L., Berry, S. H., Duan, N., Frankel, M. R., Klein, J. D., … Bozzette, S. A. (2001). The care of HIV-infected adults in rural areas of the United States. *Journal of Acquired Immune Deficiency Syndromes, 28*(4), 385–392.

Cummins, N. W., Badley, A. D., Kasten, M. J., Sampath, R., Temesgen, Z., Whitaker, J. A., … Rizza, S. A. (2016). Twenty years of human immunodeficiency virus care at the Mayo Clinic: Past, present and future. World *Journal of Virology, 5*(2), 63–67. doi:10.5501/wjv.v5.i2.63

De Cock, K. M., Jaffe, H. W., & Curran, J. W. (2011). Reflections on 30 years of AIDS. *Emerging Infectious Diseases Journal, 17*(6). doi:10.3201/eid1706.100184 (Serial on the internet).

Dillon, M., & Savage, S. (2006). Values and religion in rural America: Attitudes toward abortion and same-sex relations. *The Carsey School of Public Policy at the Scholars' Repository.* Retrieved from http://scholars.unh.edu/cgi/viewcontent.cgi?article=1011&context=carsey

Dreisbach, S. (2009). HIV/AIDS in rural America: Challenges and promising strategies. Retrieved from http://www.indiana.edu/ ~ aids/factsheets/factsheet23.pdf

Goldin, C. S. (1994). Stigmatization and AIDS: Critical issues in public health. *Social Science and Medicine, 39*(9), 1359–1366. Retrieved from http://www.ncbi.nlm.nih.gov/pubmed/7801171

Graham, R. P., Forrester, M. L., Wysong, J. A., Rosenthal, T. C., & James, P. A. (1995). HIV/AIDS in the rural United States: Epidemiology and health services delivery. *Medical Care Research and Review, 52*(4), 435–452.

Haverkos, H. W., & Curran, J. W. (1982). The current outbreak of Kaposi's sarcoma and opportunistic infections. *CA: A Cancer Journal for Clinicians, 32*(6), 330–339.

Health Resources and Services Administration. (2010). HRSA care action: Workforce capacity in HIV. Retrieved from http://hab.hrsa.gov/newspublications/careactionnewsletter/april2010.pdf

Heckman, T. G., Somlai, A. M., Kelly, J. A., Stevenson, L. Y., & Galdabini, K. (1996). Reducing barriers to care and improving quality of life for rural persons with HIV. *AIDS Patient Care STDS, 10*(1), 37–43. doi:10.1089/apc.1996.10.37

Heckman, T. G., Somlai, A. M., Peters, J., Walker, J., Otto-Salaj, L., Galdabini, C. A., & Kelly, J. A. (1998). Barriers to care among persons living with HIV/AIDS in urban and rural areas. *AIDS Care, 10*(3), 365–375. doi:10.1080/713612410

Lam, N. S., & Liu, K. B. (1994). Spread of AIDS in rural America, 1982–1990. *Journal of Acquired Immune Deficiency Syndromes, 7*(5), 485–490.

Lipka, M., & Wormald, B. (2016). How religious is your state? Retrieved from http://www.pewresearch.org/fact-tank/2016/02/29/how-religious-is-your-state/?state=alabama

McNeal, C., & Perkins, I. (2007). Potential roles of black churches in HIV/AIDS prevention. *Journal of Human Behavior in the Social Environment, 15*(2–3), 219–232.

National Institutes of Health. (2015). NIH HIV/AIDS research priorities and guidelines for determining AIDS funding. Retrieved from https://grants.nih.gov/grants/guide/notice-files/NOT-OD-15-137.html

Parker, R., & Aggleton, P. (2003). HIV and AIDS-related stigma and discrimination: A conceptual framework and implications for action. *Social Science and Medicine, 57*(1), 13–24.

Preston, D. B., D'Augelli, A. R., Kassab, C. D., Cain, R. E., Schulze, F. W., & Starks, M. T. (2004). The influence of stigma on the sexual risk behavior of rural men who have sex with men. *AIDS Education and Prevention, 16*(4), 291–303. doi:10.1521/aeap.16.4.291.40401

Reif, S., Golin, C. E., & Smith, S. R. (2005). Barriers to accessing HIV/AIDS care in North Carolina: Rural and urban differences. *AIDS Care, 17*(5), 558–565.

Rural Center for AIDS/STD Prevention. (2009). In S. Driesbach, R. A. Crosby, S. M. Noar, & W. L. Yarber (Eds.), *Tearing down fences: HIV/STD prevention in America.*

Sengupta, S., Banks, B., Jonas, D., Miles, M. S., & Smith, G. C. (2011). HIV interventions to reduce HIV/AIDS stigma: A systematic review. *AIDS and Behavior, 15*(6), 1075–1087.

Smith, J. E., Landau, J., & Bahr, G. R. (2009). AIDS in rural and small town America: Making the heartland respond. *AIDS Patient Care, 4*(3), 17–21.

Sowell, R. L., Lowenstein, A., Moneyham, L., Demi, A., Mizuno, Y., & Seals, B. F. (1997). Resources, stigma, and patterns of disclosure in rural women with HIV infection. *Public Health Nursing, 14*(5), 302–312.

The Henry J. Kaiser Family Foundation. (2016). HIV testing in the United States. Retrieved from http://kff.org/hivaids/fact-sheet/hiv-testing-in-the-united-states/

Topping, S., & Hartwig, L. C. (1997). Delivering care to rural HIV/AIDS patients. *The Journal of Rural Health, 13*(3), 226–236.

U.S. Department of Health and Human Services. (2015). *30 years of HIV/AIDS timeline*. Retrieved from https://www.aids.gov/hiv-aids-basics/hiv-aids-101/aids-timeline/

Chapter 4
HIV Medications: Why They Work and Why They Fail

Gregory S. Felzien

HIV therapy advances over the last several years have altered outcomes and changed HIV into a long-term, treatable, chronic disease. This has cultivated greater optimism and has shifted the focus of HIV therapy to one of management with a team approach to treatment. All of these advances, however, are only realized if medications are taken properly and as prescribed. Currently, there is no available cure or vaccine, therefore, it is important to know your HIV status and to prevent HIV infection and transmission through a personalized comprehensive sexual/prevention plan. It is equally important, if diagnosed with HIV, to enter into care early with an HIV provider, understand treatment regimens, follow-through with your health plan, and take medications, if prescribed, as directed.

This journey begins with understanding how the HIV virus is transmitted, enters the body, and causes lifelong infection. Knowledge of the HIV virus can minimize the transmission of the virus to others, create a greater understanding of why adherence to all aspects of care is so vital for long term, good health, and minimize the risk of being infected with a resistant strain of HIV which can affect current and future treatment options.

The HIV virus is transmitted through exposure of certain body fluids, such as blood, semen (*cum*), pre-seminal fluid (*pre-cum*), rectal fluids, vaginal fluids, and breast milk from an individual who is HIV-infected. These particular fluids transmit the HIV virus when they come into contact with mucous membranes, such as the rectum, vagina, penis, or mouth. The HIV virus can also be transmitted through damaged tissue or by being directly injected into the bloodstream. HIV is spread in the United States mainly by having anal or vaginal sex with someone who is HIV-infected without using a condom. The risk of transmitting HIV is far greater when the HIV-positive partner's HIV is not adequately controlled. HIV is also

G.S. Felzien (✉)
Georgia Department of Public Health, Division of Health Protection/IDI-HIV,
2 Peachtree St., NW, Suite 16-428, Atlanta, GA 30303-3142, USA
e-mail: gregory.felzien@dph.ga.gov

© Springer International Publishing AG 2017
F.M. Parks et al. (eds.), *HIV/AIDS in Rural Communities*,
DOI 10.1007/978-3-319-56239-1_4

45

spread by sharing needles and syringes used to prepare drugs for injection with someone who is HIV-infected. The virus can live in a used needle up to 42 days depending on temperature and other environmental factors. Less common modes of HIV transmission occur from mother to child during pregnancy, birth, or breast-feeding or by being stuck with an HIV-contaminated needle or other sharp object.

Rare cases of HIV transmission in the United States can occur with: (1) oral sex, (2) receiving blood transfusions, blood products, or organ/tissue transplants that are contaminated with HIV, (3) eating food that has been pre-chewed by an HIV-infected person, (4) being bitten by a person with HIV, (5) contact between broken skin, wounds, or mucous membranes with HIV-infected blood or blood-contaminated body fluids or (6) by deep, open-mouth kissing if both partners have sores or bleeding gums and blood from the HIV-infected person gets into the bloodstream of an HIV-negative partner. HIV is not spread through saliva (HIV Transmission, 2016; Centers for Disease Control and Prevention, n.d.).

Once the HIV virus enters the body, there are seven stages of the HIV life cycle (Fig. 4.1) which include binding, fusion, reverse transcription, integration, repli-cation, assembly, and budding. Knowledge of these stages helps in the under-standing how each of the six, currently available, classes of HIV medications work and the need to block three unique steps in the HIV life cycle in order to control HIV replication, i.e., the formation of new viruses within the body (HIV Overview, The HIV Life Cycle, 2015). Continued research has expanded upon the under-standing of HIV replication, which has opened the door for potential targets for blocking HIV viral replication and the development of new HIV therapies. For instance, research on the final step of the HIV virus life cycle (Fig. 4.1 step 7), where smaller HIV proteins combine to transform an immature (noninfectious) virus to form mature (infectious) HIV, may be a target for new classes of HIV medications. This final maturation step in the HIV life cycle is essential for HIV infectivity, otherwise any inhibition at this stage, via maturation inhibitors, leads to the production of noninfectious HIV particles (Wang, Lu, & Li, 2015).

Controlling HIV takes three medications, selected from the six current classes of HIV treatment options which affect unique pathways along the HIV life cycle. Taking these medications incorrectly or as a partial medication regimen, i.e., taking only one or two of the three prescribed medications, can result in the development of resistance to the prescribed medications and cross-resistance to medications within the same HIV medication class. Abrupt discontinuation of many medications can result in a withdrawal syndrome and could potentially be fatal. For example, if prescribed effective high blood pressure medication, stopping the medication abruptly can have harmful effects, such as an abnormal heart rhythm, chest pain, increased blood pressure, or stroke (Reidenberg, 2011). Yet, if the same medication is reinitiated, one would expect the medication to maintain its effectiveness with a drop in blood pressure. Stopping and starting HIV medications, missing doses, or taking the medications at various times throughout the day can allow the HIV virus to replicate at higher levels, resulting in it finding ways around the HIV therapy and causing the development of medication resistance and cross-resistance with ulti-mate treatment failure. This also occurs when abruptly stopping an HIV medication

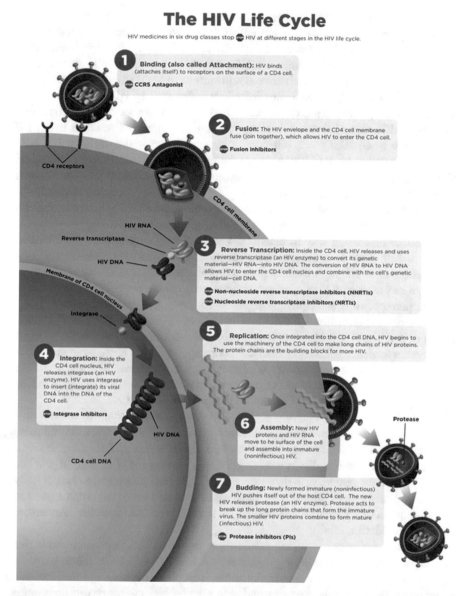

Fig. 4.1 HIV overview, The HIV life cycle (2015)

regimen in that each part of the medication regimen is metabolized, i.e., processed by the body to inactivate medications prior to elimination from the body, at different rates and can create a situation where the HIV virus is "seeing" only one or two medications. This can potentially cause more rapid development of medication resistance causing these medications to no longer work in controlling HIV replication if restarted (Management of the Treatment-Experienced Patient, 2015).

In addition to not taking medication regimens as prescribed, resistant strains of the HIV virus, which can effect current and/or future treatment options, can be transmitted to HIV-infected and HIV-uninfected individuals through unprotected sex or by sharing needles with an HIV-infected individual who has already developed HIV medication resistance (Goldsamt et al., 2011; Boden et al., 1999; Kozal et al., 2005). This secondary infection may result in HIV medications not working, although they are taken as prescribed. It can be a shock for someone who has engaged in these behaviors to discover that they are now resistant to 8 or 9 medications when taking one pill once a day, which contains three active HIV medications (What to Start, 2016), since being diagnosed and initially started on HIV therapy. So, it is important to know your and your partners' HIV status, start treatment and encourage your partner to be on appropriate treatment if HIV-infected, wear condoms with every sexual encounter, and avoid sharing needles and syringes used to prepare drugs for injection.

In further discussing why medications work and why they fail, we must look at human nature with an emphasis on adherence, teamwork, barriers, stigma, discrimination, and bridging treatment gaps to comprehend how and why medications are taken as prescribed. First, medication adherence can be defined as: adherence to (or compliance with) a medication regimen as the extent to which patients take medications as prescribed by their healthcare providers (Osterberg & Blaschke, 2005) or the extent to which a person's behavior—taking medication, following a diet, and/or executing lifestyle changes—corresponds with agreed recommendations from a healthcare provider (Adherence to Long-Term Therapies, 2003). Overall, the bottom line is; "Drugs don't work in patients who don't take them," as stated by the former Surgeon General C. Everett Koop, M.D.

When discussing and thinking about adherence, it is important to remind ourselves that we are human. Taking medications daily as prescribed is a commitment and change in our daily routine. It is, therefore, useful to set up reminders that will ensure adherence, especially as we integrate this change into our daily lives. The use of pill boxes, phone, or wristwatch alarms, pill reminder apps, setting a daily routine or placing medications in the same place each and every day, such as next to our toothbrush or TV remote, can keep us on track (Dayer, Heldenbrand, Anderson, Gubbins, & Martin, 2003).

There are challenges in taking medications as prescribed, on a daily basis, for any chronic disease. Simplifying regimens, decreasing pill and/or bottle burdens, considering food and storage requirements, stopping unnecessary medications, minimizing drug–drug interactions and side effects, and taking medications once daily are key in improving long-term daily adherence (Limitations to Treatment Safety and Efficacy, Adherence to Antiretroviral, 2014; Nachega et al., 2014).

Several studies have looked at medication adherence for a variety of chronic disease processes, which demonstrated rapid drop-offs in not only taking, but filling prescriptions on a regular basis (Fig. 4.2). Poor adherence causes approximately 33–69% of medication-related hospitalizations and accounts for $100 billion in annual healthcare costs (Osterberg & Blaschke, 2005). Therefore, asking questions, understanding why medications are prescribed, understanding and minimizing

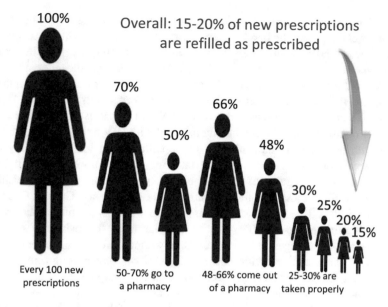

Fig. 4.2 Based on IMS health data (*Pharmacies* improving health, reducing costs, 2011)

potential side effects, and discussing ways to reduce the number of medications taken daily are all important for good health and long-term adherence to treatment.

Being diagnosed with any chronic disease is challenging, but understanding the disease and what measures need to be taken to control it are empowering. Although the current HIV guidelines recommend therapy for all HIV-infected individuals in reducing morbidity, mortality and preventing HIV transmission, regardless of CD4 cell count levels, it is important to have an understanding of the benefits of treatment and address strategies to optimize adherence. On a case-by-case basis, HIV therapy may be deferred due to clinical and/or psychosocial factors, but should be initiated as soon as possible (Initiation of Antiretroviral Therapy, 2016). The goal is education with a full understanding of the benefits of treatment and what it means to live with and be on HIV therapy. Be Ready.

Another important factor to consider in discussing why medications work and why they fail is stigma and discrimination. Having been diagnosed with HIV, educating ourselves, deciding we are ready for medications, and now having a prescription in hand for HIV therapy—we are in charge, but now what? If all concerns are not discussed prior to starting HIV treatment the mind may start to race with thoughts of will someone at the pharmacy know me and tell everyone about my HIV, can I really do this, will I have side effects, what kind of additional stigma and discrimination will I face, are there state laws if I do not tell my partner about my HIV and they become infected?

There are, in many states, active laws concerning testing and disclosure of HIV (State HIV Laws, 2015; State Criminal Statutes on HIV Transmission, 2008). For instance, individuals may be guilty of a felony and, upon conviction, shall be punished by imprisonment for up to ten years through reckless conduct causing harm to or endangering the bodily safety of another individual. This occurs through conduct by an HIV-infected person or assault by an HIV- or hepatitis-infected person who knowingly engages in an act (sexual, sharing needles, donating blood or tissue) and the HIV-infected person does not disclose to the other person the fact of being an HIV- or hepatitis-infected person prior to engaging in said act. This law goes on to state that if a person who is an HIV—or hepatitis-infected person and who, after obtaining knowledge of being infected with HIV or hepatitis, commits an assault with the intent to transmit HIV or hepatitis, using his or her body fluids (blood, semen, or vaginal secretions), saliva, urine, or feces upon: a peace officer or a correctional officer is guilty of a felony and, upon conviction, shall be punished by imprisonment for not less than five nor more than twenty years (Georgia Code O.C. G.A. § 16-5-60, 2015). Other states comment that it is unlawful for any person, knowing him/herself to be HIV positive and knowing the risk of transmission through sexual intercourse, to have intercourse without informing his/her partner of his/her HIV status and receiving consent. In addition, any person who, knowing him/herself to be HIV positive and knowing that HIV may be transmitted through donating blood, plasma, organs, skin, or other human tissue, donates blood, plasma, organs, skin, or other human tissue is guilty of a felony of the third degree. A third-degree felony is punishable up to five years (The 2016 Florida Statutes, PUBLIC HEALTH, Chapter 384, 2016; The 2016 Florida Statutes, PUBLIC HEALTH, Chapter 381, 2016). These types of laws can potentially create barriers, add to stigma and discrimination and, as some individuals and groups support, require updates and changes in order to minimize these barriers. It is important to understand current laws and regulations within the state you reside. Still, this should not detour the need for creating a support system, as support for those individuals with chronic diseases enhances adherence and improves care (Scheurer, Choudhry, Swanton, Matlin, & Shrank, 2012; Poudel, Buchanan, Amiya, Poudel-Tandukar, 2015).

Knowing the applicable laws in your area is the first step in developing trust in the treatment process. A thorough understanding of an individual's specific needs is vital in overcoming real and perceived barriers, yet questions still may arise about stigma and discrimination that influence access to the prescribed medication: what pharmacy am I going to use, will I know someone there, are they going to tell others in the community about my HIV, and/or should I travel to another town, city or county to obtain my HIV medications? This is a multifaceted process in considering what works best for each individual and situation. Factors to consider before starting medications may include:

Transportation: How am I going to get to the pharmacy; how can I minimize the number of times I go to the pharmacy; can I get my medications mailed to me, and if so, how do I prevent others in the home from seeing my medication when they are delivered; and do I need to go to a pharmacy in another county in order to minimize the risk of someone finding out I have HIV? This is an individual decision in that one solution does not fit all in deciding what would work best in each situation. This is where a strong case manager to patient relationship is of great benefit in discussing and thinking through the process prior to receiving a prescription for HIV medications. Be ready and know what to ask when getting to this point in understanding any issues with the AIDS Drug Assistance Program (ADAP), insurance medication co-pays, or other insurance requirements, such as picking up medications at certain pharmacies or being required to use mail order systems.

HIPAA: Understanding that the Health Insurance Portability and Accountability Act (HIPAA) is in effect at all levels of health care and gives rights over health information and sets rules and limits on who can look at and receive health information. In addition, HIPAA applies to all forms of an individuals' protected health information, whether electronic, written, or oral. Health insurance companies, healthcare providers, and individuals receiving care have access to healthcare records. HIPAA was established to protect the client even within settings, where individuals at the local pharmacy, especially in rural areas, are those you attended school with, go to church with, work with their family, etc. Therefore, if one's rights are being denied or health information is not being protected, there are avenues to take action with the U.S. Department of Health and Human Services (U.S. Department of Health & Human Services, Summary of the HIPAA Privacy Rule, n.d.; U.S. Department of Health & Human Services, How to File a Health Information Privacy or Security Complaint, n.d.).

Privacy: Following a diagnosis of HIV, an individual may not want to disclose their status to others and will go to great lengths to hide medications and educational material due to concerns of becoming isolated, if these items are discovered, from family and friends, stigma, and discrimination. Therefore, when discussing treatment options, make sure that the HIV treatment regimen is as simple as possible, can potentially fit in a keychain pillbox, and does not require that medications be in two separate places, such as when one medication requires refrigeration and others do not. If there is a concern of someone discovering educational material, such as flyers, brochures, etc., then ask for a list of reputable websites to find reliable information, i.e., www.cdc.gov/hiv/, hivinsite.ucsf.edu, www.aidsinfonet. org/, aidsinfo.nih.gov/guidelines, www.aids.gov, etc. Avoid blogs that are used as "pick-up" sites in that many comments are made by individuals without a full understanding of HIV and may offer inaccurate advice in order to "hook-up". Be ready, be safe, and be knowledgeable.

Family: Define what family means to you. Definitions may include a household, clan, race, fellowship and may include those that are typically considered extended family (Merriam-Webster Dictionary, Family, n.d.; Merriam-Webster Dictionary, Extended Family, n.d.). Many times, family is typically thought of as spouse, partner, mother, father, sisters, brothers, and, in close knit families, grandparents, aunts, uncles, cousins, etc. Yet we must consider individuals and groups where we spend a lot of our time, as part of our extended family. This may include those we interact with at work, faith-based organizations, close friends, etc. With any long-term life event, such as HIV care, it is important to draw on these resources for support and insight in order to maintain good health—physically, spiritually, emotionally, and mentally. Therefore, how do we draw on this support network while living with HIV? Isolating ourselves can be detrimental to all aspects of our lives with reports of suicide from feeling isolated from the world (Shittu et al., 2014; Suicidality and Violence in Patients with HIV/AIDS, 2007). First, one is not legally bound to tell family, friends, bosses, etc. about being HIV positive. Yet, there are circumstances, depending on local laws, where there are potential legal repercussions concerning disclosing one's status to those that may be at risk of acquiring HIV, such as sexual partners, sharing needles, donating blood, etc. So, how do we tell someone about our HIV status in order to develop this necessary support network? There are several things that must be considered before deciding to tell people about their HIV status:

- Think about the people you rely on for support, like family, friends, or coworkers.
- What kind of relationship do you have with these people?
- What are the pros and cons of telling them you are living with HIV?
- Are there any issues they might have that will affect how much they can support you?
- What is that person's attitude and knowledge about HIV?
- Why exactly do you want to disclose to this person?
- What kind of support can this person provide?
- For each person, ask yourself if the person needs to know now—or is it better to wait.

Once you have decided to disclose your HIV status to someone, there are a few things that can help in this endeavor, but keep in mind each person and situation may require different approaches. Having HIV does not mean that you are unlovable, do not deserve to be in a relationship, do not have the right to get married, have children, get an education, have a good job, be promoted, and above all, in getting the support that you need and deserve. When deciding to disclose HIV to someone, think it through, take it slow, and then proceed only when you are ready. Remember, you are the one in control. A few tips when disclosing your HIV status are as follows (Start Talking. Stop HIV, 2016; DO YOU HAVE TO TELL?, 2009; Telling Others You are HIV Positive, 2014);

- Be strong and confident in who you are!
- Be honest and respectful to yourself and to those you are telling.
- Educate yourself and be ready for questions. Remember, you do not have to have all the answers.
- Stick to the facts about HIV by using a reputable website for reference and avoid myths.
- Keep the first discussion short and focus on why you are telling this person.
- Talk about your status earlier in the relationship rather than later.
- Do not wait until the heat of the moment to start talking about HIV.
- Do not force the conversation. Find the right time and place for the discussion.
- Pick a safe place, if possible, bring someone with you that already knows your status.

- Do not just talk one time, have periodic conversations.
- Use multiple methods. Not every conversation has to be detailed or face to face.
- Above all—Be Safe. Be prepared to walk away if the discussion turns "ugly".

Paying for medication(s): Paying for medications should not break the bank. Know all available options and minimize any potential surprises as HIV medications have an upward cost of $3000 per month (Limitations to Treatment Safety and Efficacy, Cost Considerations and Antiretroviral Therapy, 2015), and paying out of pocket is not realistic. Understanding all of the available options in paying for these medications is important and will minimize gaps in therapy when obtaining/losing insurance or having high medication, out of pocket, co-pays. This is where having a good relationship with the case manager is imperative so that these questions can be asked early in the process without assumptions resulting in not being able to obtain and/or consistently take medications. In addition, calling the case manager early if one loses, changes, or obtains insurance coverage will enable them to access the appropriate programs and minimize gaps in services. Calling the day of taking your last pill and assuming the clinic has medications available on-site will result in gaps in taking medication properly and may result in the development of resistance to some medications. Do not fall into this trap! Medication assistance programs include;

- AIDS Drug Assistance Program (ADAP): http://hab.hrsa.gov/abouthab/partbdrug.html.
- Co-pay cards: If qualified, assists with medication co-pay costs with certain insurance.
- Pharmaceutical Assistance Program (PAP): Some pharmaceutical companies offer assistance programs for the drugs they manufacture and can be located at www.medicare.gov/pharmaceutical-assistance-program/ or www.rxassist.org/.
- National programs to assist based on certain disease processes, such as the HealthWell Foundation (www.healthwellfoundation.org) or the Patient Advocate Foundation (www.copays.org).
- Non-HIV medications: There are free services that can assist in saving up to 80% of the cost of non-HIV medications. These programs, such as Goodrx (www.goodrx.com/) or Needymeds (www.needymeds.com/), can decrease monthly pharmacy bills, which may assist in decreasing gaps in services due to financial constraints.

Proactively managing your HIV is a challenging, yet achievable, system of events in maintaining adherence, remaining in care and keeping HIV under control. It requires a multidisciplinary team approach that includes, most importantly, the individual with HIV and the support network, which includes family, friends, and the HIV clinic, providers, and pharmacies. Therefore, how can these medications be better managed, kept on track, and where does the HIV care team fit into this process?

The use of a multidisciplinary team approach can provide an accessible, trustworthy healthcare system that focuses on and creates a nonjudgmental environment.

Keys to promoting such an environment are the responsibility of the entire team, including providers, support networks and the individual with HIV. Items that your treatment team should address include:

- Following the diagnosis of HIV, promoting early linkage to and retention in HIV care.
- Promoting strong, positive relationships within a multidisciplinary team.
- Promoting involvement of friends, family, etc., as soon as possible, in the process.
- Having open, two-way discussions on readiness to start daily medications.
- Involving everyone in the HIV medication selection, not just the providers.
- Seeking reliable information about HIV disease, prevention, and treatment.
- Identifying potential barriers to adherence, and necessary medication management skills.
- Being cognizant of beliefs, perceptions, expectations, life schedules, language, and literacy.
- Providing medication coverage, stable housing, social support, and income and food security.
- Assessing needs for other medical conditions, mental health, and psychosocial factors.
- Assessing adherence at every clinic visit and maintaining open communication in discussing barriers.
- Being open and positive in discussing adherence success and barriers.
- Identifying the type of and reasons for adherence barriers and set reasonable goals for success.
- Monitoring retention in care and reaching out to those patients that are unable to keep appointments or who drop out of care.
- Limitations to Treatment Safety and Efficacy, Adherence to Antiretroviral, 2014.

Recognize that human nature plays a major role in this process and that good communication is a two-way street. Be an active part of the treatment plan. Sitting idly by, nodding your head and accepting what the provider is recommending can create misunderstanding and a barrier to good health. Prior to starting treatment, make sure there is a clear understanding of the treatment program, any personal and logistical obstacles to adhering to the treatment plan have been addressed and you are prepared to take medications, as prescribed, on a daily basis. Additional conversations may be warranted with the provider, case manager, friends, family, or support network prior to receiving a prescription for HIV medications. There may be situations where waiting to begin HIV medications is the right choice. Having open communication with the treatment team is imperative in that stopping treatment on your own or taking a treatment regimen incorrectly can result in the development of resistance to the prescribed HIV medication regimen.

Great strides in HIV therapy have been taken in recent years. HIV is a treatable, chronic disease and there is much reason for optimism if medications are taken properly and as prescribed. This is an achievable endeavor and possible when you take charge of yourself and your health. There is currently no vaccine or cure for HIV, but with advancements in treatment, we have seen life expectancy increase from 36.1 to 51.4 years from 2000–2002 to 2006–2007. In general, a 20-year-old HIV-positive adult on HIV medications in the United States or Canada is expected to live into their early 70s, a life expectancy approaching that of the general population. Still, this life expectancy can be decreased due to other factors, such as smoking, and should be discussed as part of a comprehensive health plan (Samji et al., 2013; Helleberg et al., 2015).

Therefore, find an HIV expert, stay in close contact with your providers, remember you are an integral part of the treatment team, discuss any natural therapies in that they could be helpful/harmful to your overall health, and look for inner and external support during this journey.

Be Safe. Be Smart. Be an Active Part of Your Individual Journey.

References

Adherence to Long-Term Therapies - Evidence for Action. (2003). Retrieved from http://apps.who.int/medicinedocs/en/d/Js4883e/6.html

Boden, D., Hurley, A., Zhang, L., Cao, Y., Guo, Y., Jones, E., Tsay, J., Ip, J., Farthing, C., Limoli, K., Parkin, N., & Markowitz, M. (1999). HIV-1 drug resistance in newly infected individuals. *The Journal of the American Medical Association, 282*(12), 1135–1141.

Centers for Disease Control and Prevention. (n.d.). HIV Risk Reduction Tool. Retrieved from http://wwwn.cdc.gov/hivrisk/estimator.html

Dayer, L., Heldenbrand, S., Anderson, P., Gubbins, P. O., & Martin, B. C. (2003). Smartphone medication adherence apps: Potential benefits to patients and providers. *Journal of the American Pharmacists Association, 53*(2), 172–181.

DO YOU HAVE TO TELL?, Sharing Your HIV Status. (2009). Retrieved from https://www.aids.gov/hiv-aids-basics/just-diagnosed-with-hiv-aids/talking-about-your-status/do-you-have-to-tell/

Georgia Code O.C.G.A. § 16-5-60. (2015). Retrieved from http://www.legis.ga.gov/en-US/default.aspx

Goldsamt, L. A., Clatts, M. C., Parker, M. M., Colon, V., Hallack, R., & Messina, M. G. (2011). Prevalence of sexually acquired antiretroviral drug resistance in a community sample of HIV-Positive men who have sex with men in New York City. *AIDS Patient Care and STDS, 25*(5), 287–293.

Helleberg, M., May, M. T., Ingle, S. M., Dabis, F., Reiss, P., Fätkenheuer, G., ..., Obela, N. (2015). Smoking and life expectancy among HIV-infected individuals on antiretroviral therapy in Europe and North America. *AIDS, 29*(2), 221–229.

HIV Overview, The HIV Life Cycle. (2015). Retrieved from https://aidsinfo.nih.gov/education-materials/fact-sheets/19/73/the-hiv-life-cycle. Accessed July 15, 2016.

HIV Transmission. (2016). Retrieved from http://www.cdc.gov/hiv/basics/transmission.html

Initiation of Antiretroviral Therapy. (2016). Retrieved from https://aidsinfo.nih.gov/guidelines/html/1/adult-and-adolescent-arv-guidelines/10/initiation-of-antiretroviral-therapy

Kozal, M. J., Amico, K. R., Chiarella, J., Cornman, D., Fisher, W., Fisher, J., et al. (2005). HIV drug resistance and HIV transmission risk behaviors among active injection drug users. *Journal of Acquired Immune Deficiency Syndromes, 40*(1), 106–109.

Limitations to Treatment Safety and Efficacy, Adherence to Antiretroviral. (2014). Retrieved from https://aidsinfo.nih.gov/guidelines/html/1/adult-and-adolescent-arv-guidelines/30/adherence-to-art

Limitations to Treatment Safety and Efficacy, Cost Considerations and Antiretroviral Therapy. (2015). Retrieved from https://aidsinfo.nih.gov/guidelines/html/1/adult-and-adolescent-arv-guidelines/459/cost-considerations-and-antiretroviral-therapy

Management of the Treatment-Experienced Patient, Discontinuation or Interruption of Antiretroviral Therapy. (2015). Received from https://aidsinfo.nih.gov/guidelines/html/1/adult-and-adolescent-arv-guidelines/18/discontinuation-or-interruption-of-antiretroviral-therapy

Merriam-Webster Dictionary. (n.d.). Family. Retrieved from http://www.merriam-webster.com/dictionary/family

Merriam-Webster Dictionary. (n.d.). Extended family. Retrieved from http://www.merriam-webster.com/dictionary/extended%20family

Nachega, J. B., Parienti, J. J., Uthman, O. A., Gross, R., Dowdy, D. W., Sax, P. E., ..., Giordano, T.P. (2014). Lower Pill Burden and once-daily dosing antiretroviral treatment regimens for hiv infection: Meta-Analysis of randomized controlled trials. *Clinical Infectious Diseases, 58*(9), 1297–1307.

Osterberg, L., & Blaschke, T. (2005). Adherence to medications. *The New England Journal of Medicine, 353,* 487–497.

Pharmacies: Improving Health, Reducing Costs. (2011). Retrieved from http://www.nacds.org/pdfs/pr/2011/PrinciplesOfHealthcare.pdf

Poudel, K. C., Buchanan, D. R., Amiya, R. M., & Poudel-Tandukar, K. (2015). Perceived family support and antiretroviral adherence in HIV-Positive individuals: Results from a community-based positive living with HIV study. *International Quarterly of Community Health Education, 36*(1), 71–91.

Reidenberg, M. M. (2011). Drug discontinuation effects are part of the pharmacology of a drug. *The Journal of Pharmacology And Experimental Therapeutics, 339*(2), 324–328.

Samji, H., Cescon, A., Hogg, R. S., Modur, S. P., Althoff, K. N., Buchacz, K., ..., Gange, S. J. (2013). Closing the gap: Increases in life expectancy among treated HIV-positive individuals in the United States and Canada. *PLoS ONE, 8*(12), e81355.

Scheurer, D., Choudhry, N., Swanton, K. A., Matlin, O., & Shrank, W. (2012). Association between different types of social support and medication adherence. *The American Journal of Managed Care, 18*(12), e461–e467.

Shittu, R. O., Alabi, M. K., Odeigah, L. O., Sanni, M. A., Issa, B. A., Olanrewaju, A. T., ..., Aderibigbe, S.A. (2014). Suicidal ideation among depressed people living with HIV/AIDS in Nigeria, West Africa. *Open Journal of Medical Psychology, 3,* 262–270.

Start Talking. Stop HIV. (2016). Retrieved from http://www.cdc.gov/actagainstaids/campaigns/starttalking/index.html

STATE CRIMINAL STATUTES ON HIV TRANSMISSION. (2008). Retrieved from https://www.aclu.org/state-criminal-statutes-hiv-transmission?redirect=lgbt-rights_hiv-aids/state-criminal-statutes-hiv-transmission

State HIV Laws. (2015). Retrieved from http://www.cdc.gov/hiv/policies/law/states/index.html

Suicidality and Violence in Patients with HIV/AIDS. (2007). Retrieved from http://www.hivguidelines.org/clinical-guidelines/hiv-and-mental-health/suicidality-and-violence-in-patients-with-hivaids/

Telling Others You are HIV Positive. (2014). Retrieved from http://www.aidsinfonet.org/fact_sheets/view/204

The 2016 Florida Statutes, PUBLIC HEALTH, Chapter 381, PUBLIC HEALTH: GENERAL PROVISIONS. (2016). Retrieved from http://www.leg.state.fl.us/statutes/index.cfm?mode=View%20Statutes&SubMenu=1&App_mode=Display_Statute&Search_String=381.0041&URL=0300-0399/0381/Sections/0381.0041.html

The 2016 Florida Statutes, PUBLIC HEALTH, Chapter 384, SEXUALLY TRANSMISSIBLE
     DISEASES. (2016). Retrieved from http://www.leg.state.fl.us/Statutes/index.cfm?App_mode=
     Display_Statute&Search_String=&URL=0300-0399/0384/Sections/0384.34.html
U.S. Department of Health & Human Services. (n.d.). How to file a health information privacy or
     security complaint. Retrieved from http://www.hhs.gov/hipaa/filing-a-complaint/complaint-
     process/index.html
U.S. Department of Health & Human Services. (n.d.). Summary of the HIPAA privacy rule.
     Retrieved from http://www.hhs.gov/hipaa/for-professionals/privacy/laws-regulations/
Wang, D., Lu, W., & Li, F. (2015). Pharmacological intervention of HIV-1 maturation. *Acta
     Pharmaceutica Sinica B, 5*(6), 493–499.
What to Start: Initial Combination Regimens for the Antiretroviral-Naive Patient. (2016).
     Retrieved from https://aidsinfo.nih.gov/guidelines/html/1/adult-and-adolescent-arv-guidelines/
     11/what-to-start

Chapter 5
HIV Prevention: Treatment as Prevention (TasP), Occupational Postexposure Prophylaxis (oPEP), Nonoccupational Postexposure Prophylaxis (nPEP), and Pre-exposure Prophylaxis (PrEP)

Neal A. Carnes, John Malone and Jordan Helms

Introduction: A Brief History of HIV Prevention in the U.S.

On June 5, 1981 the now Centers for Disease Control and Prevention (CDC) published a seminal report of a rare lung infection, *Pneumocystis carinii pneumonia* (PCP), diagnosed in five men living in Los Angeles, California (CDC, 1981). The initial five cases were notable given they occurred in young, otherwise healthy gay men, and PCP more often occurs in people with compromised immune systems, such as the elderly. At the time of the report, no one could predict these men were to become index cases of a disease that would challenge and redefine medical and social response systems, as well as decimate generations within particular communities. Tragically, all five of the initial cases died from a disease we would come to know as Acquired Immune Deficiency Syndrome (AIDS).

Since 1981, the World Health Organization (WHO, n.d.) estimates 79 million people have been infected with HIV, the causal agent to AIDS. Of the estimated 79 million people infected since 1981, 39 million are believed to have died and another 1.2 million die annually. To put this death count in perspective, every year the population of Dallas, Texas (the 9th largest city in the U.S.) succumbs to HIV.

N.A. Carnes
Georgia State University, Atlanta, USA
e-mail: ncarnes2@student.gsu.edu

J. Malone
Georgia Department of Public Health, Atlanta, USA
e-mail: john.malone@dph.ga.gov

J. Helms (✉)
Emory University—Rollins School of Public Health, Atlanta, USA
e-mail: Jordan.helms@emory.edu

© Springer International Publishing AG 2017
F.M. Parks et al. (eds.), *HIV/AIDS in Rural Communities*,
DOI 10.1007/978-3-319-56239-1_5

In the United States, the CDC estimates approximately 1.2 million people are living with HIV, between 40,000 and 50,000 become infected each year, and nearly 700,000 people diagnosed with HIV have died (amfAR, 2016; CDC, 2016a). In 2013, 3.7% ($n = 1738$) of newly diagnosed cases and 6.2% of prevalence (total living cases) are among people living in nonmetropolitan areas, i.e., with less than 50,000 people, and another 13.8% ($n = 6456$) of newly diagnosed and 10.3% of prevalence live in areas with 50,000 to 500,000 people, aka suburban areas (CDC, n.d.; National Rural Health Association, n.d.). These rates demonstrate rural and suburban areas are less likely to house people living with HIV—regional variations exist regarding the rural-suburban-urban proportions (Hall, Lee, & McKenna, 2005). Regardless of geographical variation, studies have shown the context of rural and suburban life uniquely impacts access to and provision of prevention as well as treatment and care services (Kempf et al., 2010; Ohl & Perencevich, 2011; Sutton, Anthony, Vila, McLellan-Lemal, & Weidle, 2010). Accessibility and acceptability of services are essential to curbing the epidemic.

In this chapter, we explore four biomedical interventions that can and are reducing the number of new HIV diagnoses: TasP, oPEP), nPEP, and PrEP. The essential component to prevention interventions, including the four discussed in this chapter, is conducting a comprehensive prevention plan, e.g., discussing abstinence, condom (male and female) use, consistent testing, and promoting resiliency factors that mitigate risk behaviors. The impact these interventions, especially, when couched within comprehensive prevention planning, can have on HIV infection as well as disease progression can be quite significant and revolutionary if these tools are made readily accessible and are embraced by those engaged in risk behaviors. We begin this review by briefly exploring trends in HIV epidemiology, followed by a review of prevention, treatment, and some of the challenges to biomedical interventions.

The Current State of Affairs: An Epidemiological Profile of HIV in the U.S

Between 2005 and 2014, a number of important and laudable trends have occurred in HIV. Nationally, we have seen significant reductions in newly diagnosed cases (CDC, 2016a). For instance, 19% fewer new diagnoses occurred in 2014 compared to 2005. The most dramatic decreases were seen among those who reported injection drug use as their risk behavior (63%)[1] followed by African American

---

[1]The 2015 HIV outbreak in Austin, Indiana (a town of ~4000) and pervasively high rates of prescription drug abuse suggests this trend may not hold (O'Malley, 2015).

women (42%).[2] Across nearly all measured groups trends in newly diagnosed HIV cases are declining. This trend can be enhanced and reinforced by the prevention modalities discussed in this chapter.

Where downward trends have not been seen is among gay, bisexual, and other men who have sex with men (herein referred as to MSM), especially MSM of color. Between 2005 and 2014, MSM saw a 6% increase in new diagnoses. When looking at racial disparities within MSM communities, African American MSM experienced a 22% increase during this period, and Hispanic/Latino MSM experienced a 24% increase (CDC, 2016a). At the beginning of 2016, the CDC noted the lifetime risk for acquiring HIV is 1 in 2 among African American MSM, 1 in 4 among Latino MSM, and 1 in 11 among White MSM (CDC, 2016b). In other words, if we do nothing different or differently, 50, 25%, and approximately 10% of each respective group is likely to be living with HIV at their time of death. These rates concern rural America for while a smaller proportion of MSM are estimated to live in areas of less than 50,000 residents (Lieb et al., 2009), they live in these areas nonetheless.

Additional concerns regarding geography and HIV/AIDS also emerge. The situation for rural America is increasingly disheartening given the disproportionate impact unfolding in the Southeastern corridor of the U.S. (CDC, 2015a). The South[3] is home to slightly less than half of all HIV cases (44%), yet only a third (37%) of the nation's population (CDC, 2015a). Narrowing this lens, Georgia ranks 5th in the nation in HIV prevalence (Georgia Department of Public Health n.d. a), and second in newly diagnosed cases (Fulton County Task Force on HIV/AIDS, 2015). While the lion's share of cases reside in and around Fulton County (Atlanta), when compared to other regions, a larger portion of cases in the South reside in rural/suburban areas (Georgia Department of Public Health, n.d. b; CDC, 2016b). In sum, rural areas will not be spared ongoing concerns with HIV/AIDS given the disparity of rates in the rural South, especially among MSM.

A key concern regarding the South's disproportionate rate of HIV is the disparate rate of poverty among southerners (Adimora, Ramirez, Schoenbach, & Cohen, 2014; CDC, 2016b; Reif et al., 2014). Indeed, poverty is disproportionately concentrated in rural sections of the country, especially the South (U.S. Department of Agriculture, 2015), impacting access to consistent primary and secondary HIV prevention (Denning & DiNenno, 2015). In addition to poverty, stigma also presents concerns for HIV-related issues for rural areas (Preston et al., 2004; Sowell et al., 1997; Yannessa, Reece, & Basta, 2008). Rural area's close-knit context, fosters a great deal of concern for disclosing stigmatized identities, such as living

---

[2]Even with the decline in their rate over the prior decade, African American women remain disproportionately impacted compared to women of other racial backgrounds (60% of women's HIV cases are African-American) (CDC, 2016a).

[3]Texas, Oklahoma, Missouri, Louisiana, Mississippi, Alabama, Tennessee, Kentucky, Georgia, Florida, North and South Carolina, Virginia, Maryland, West Virginia and Delaware.

with HIV, being gay, or perceived as "sexually permissive." These factors collectively paint a picture on how best to address being at risk for as well as living with HIV in rural areas, especially in the south.

HIV Prevention in Rural Communities

Persons who live in rural areas face unique access barriers to HIV services not experienced by their metropolitan residing counterparts. For instance, rural residents often experience longer distances with few to no public transportation systems to access prevention and treatment services, there are often fewer resources, as well as less trained medical providers (Heckman et al., 1998; Reif et al., 2005). In support of the provider barrier assertion, a 2013 study conducted by the South Carolina Rural Health Research Center examined 28 states and found that 95% of rural counties lacked Ryan White-funded medical providers—those who would ensure access and adherence to effective HIV treatment (Vyavaharkar et al., 2013). In addition, rural communities are often characterized by condensed networks, where more conservative perspectives are valued, thus more stigma surrounds HIV risk groups and the behaviors related to infection (Heckman et al., 1998; Reif, Golan, & Smith, 1998; Reif et al., 2005). Each of the aforementioned aspects of rural life contributes to HIV risk and disease progression, as well as reduced healthcare quality and access (HIV/AIDS in Rural America: Challenges and Promising Strategies 2009). This context presents challenges for the implementation of the following biomedical interventions in that they require access to trained medical providers, sometimes ongoing access, and in a supportive environment, rather than a judgmental one.

Treatment as Prevention (TasP)

Approximately 15 years after the discovery of HIV/AIDS, pharmacological (aka biomedical) interventions grew in volume to the point we could consider treating those living with the disease with more than one drug. By 1995/96, seven drugs had been approved by the Food and Drug Administration (FDA) to treat HIV. At the time, we understood no single drug controlled the virus for an extended period or at an efficacious level that altered the death sentence trajectory of an HIV diagnosis. With enough drugs on the market and preliminary evidence to suggest effectiveness, researchers theorized that a combination of medications, three specifically, would be more effective in battling HIV than a lone medication; this approach to treatment was coined "(combination) antiretroviral therapy (ART)."

By the end of 1996, ART's impact was staggering and celebratory; morbidity of and mortality from advanced stage HIV (aka AIDS) was drastically reduced (Palella et al., 1998). Over the proceeding decade our knowledge of ART's effect suggested treating HIV to the point of viral suppression (not enough virus is present in blood to be detected) can prevent infections. Montaner et al. (2006) assert the research among sero-discordant couples, where the HIV negative partner remained uninfected in context to having an HIV infected partner who was prescribed ART (Gilliam et al., 1997; Quinn et al., 2000), as well as the use of HIV medications to mitigate mother-to-child transmission (Connor et al., 1994), as sound rationales to expand access to treatment to not only better control disease progression, but mediate the possibility of infection during risk encounters, e.g., needle sharing and/or unprotected sex. The theory was that treatment would reduce the amount of virus to the point an infected person becomes noninfectious. This does not mean treatment cures HIV—there is no cure at present—yet it does minimize the virus to an undetectable level, and at a level that minimizes one's ability to infect another person.

TasP underwent formal testing beginning in 2005, when the HIV Prevention Trials Network (HTPN) rolled out a pilot project: HTPN 052. In this pilot, 1763 sero-discordant couples, mostly heterosexual, were recruited across 4 continents, Africa, Asia, and North and South America (Cohen, McCauley, & Gamble, 2012). The study compared HIV infection rates among couples where the partner living with HIV was provided treatment upon enrollment (early treatment group) to couples where the infected partner was treated upon an AIDS diagnosis (delayed treatment group—the standard point of treatment initiation in 2005). As of 2011, 39 negative partners had become infected with only one of the 39 in a relationship with a person in the early treatment group (Cohen, McCauley, & Gamble, 2011). This finding strongly suggests that treating HIV also reduces the chance the infected person will pass on their infection. The authors state, "The early initiation of antiretroviral therapy reduced the rates of sexual transmission of HIV-1 and clinical events, indicating both personal and public health benefits from such therapy," (p. 493). Across various trials, TasP is estimated to reduce the chance of transmitting HIV by 96% (AVERT, 2016).

A number of concerns surround TasP as a primary prevention (keeping the uninfected from getting infected) modality, such as access to ART among the poor, the rural, as well as the importance of adherence to achieve viral suppression. Another factor capping TasP's potential is that it does not eliminate an important mode of exposure—risk engaged with someone who does not know they are infected. To be effective, TasP requires that the infected know their status, be engaged in care, prescribed ART, be adherent to ART and ultimately, they must achieve sustained viral suppression. As such, TasP should be one of several interventions available and offered during comprehensive prevention planning. Such planning is essential given all HIV pharmacological-based interventions do not prevent other diseases, such as syphilis, gonorrhea, and chlamydia, which impact susceptibility to HIV.

Occupational Postexposure Prophylaxis (oPEP)

Early on we knew next to nothing about how HIV was transmitted. We only knew that the associated illnesses were fatal in nearly all cases. Deaths were playing out in homes and hospitals for hundreds, then thousands, then tens of thousands, then hundreds of thousands of people. In the days before public health mapped HIV's epidemiological triangle, and medicine was able to develop effective treatments, healthcare providers and caretakers were called to treat the sick and dying. The brave few relied on what little knowledge was available, often not knowing if they were putting themselves at risk through the very acts of care they provided. It was not until 1983 that we deduced HIV was being transmitted through certain bodily fluids, and mainly under certain conditions, e.g., during sex and needle sharing. That same year the CDC issued the first guidelines to prevent occupational exposure among healthcare providers and caretakers, e.g., wearing gloves and other protective gear.

Seven years later, in 1990, following anecdotal evidence provided by healthcare institutions as well as a CDC surveillance project, the Public Health Service issued guidelines regarding on-the-job HIV exposures. These guidelines included the recommendation to treat exposures with the medication, zidovudine, aka AZT (CDC, 1990). This approach to preventing infection was known as postexposure prophylaxis, or PEP (Kumar, 2008). Since 1990, occupational exposure guidelines in the United States have been updated several times, and they always include oPEP as a key recommendation; in 2013, the World Health Organizations also included oPEP in their exposure guidelines (Kaplan et al., 2015).

Since introducing oPEP, dozens of new anti-HIV medications have been approved by the FDA, effectively expanding oPEP's candidate options as well as providing for more complex treatment regimens (i.e., using ART). At present, oPEP involves a 28-day course of two to three-drugs (the latter is preferred), initiated immediately to within 72 hours after an exposure (Kaplan et al., 2015). An occupational exposure is extremely concerning and should be addressed as soon as possible, preferably within hours of exposure

As with any medication there are side effects. Yet, most oPEP users report few to no side effects and of those that do report "adverse events," minor concerns such as diarrhea and nausea are the most common (Schreiner et al., 2013). In addition, and as with any intervention, oPEP is not 100% effective. Table 5.1 shows the number of reported occupational exposures as well as resulting HIV cases among healthcare providers from 1981 to 2010. The CDC reports (2011) that most of the resulting cases occurred prior to the use of ART (a three-drug combination), thus before 1996.

Nonoccupational Postexposure Prophylaxis (nPEP)

PEP's success in preventing occupational exposures produced a sound theoretical foundation for the use of pharmacological interventions, i.e., medications, to prevent HIV infection in nonoccupational settings. nPEP is the counterpart to oPEP, yet as applied to sex, injection drug, or other risk behaviors that occur outside the work environment (thus, most exposures). nPEP is a 28-day course of three antiretroviral medications which must begin within 72 hours of an exposure.

Table 5.1 Healthcare Personnel with Documented and Possible Occupationally Acquired HIV Infection, by Occupation, 1981–2010

Occupation	Documented	Possible (exposures)
Nurse	24	36
Laboratory worker, clinical	16	17
Physician, nonsurgical	6	13
Laboratory technician, nonclinical	3	–
Housekeeper/maintenance worker	2	14
Technician, surgical	2	2
Embalmer/morgue technician	1	2
Health aide/attendant	1	15
Respiratory therapist	1	2
Technician, dialysis	1	3
Dental worker, including dentist	–	6
Emergency medical technician/paramedic	–	12
Physician, surgical	–	6
Other technician/therapist	–	9
Other healthcare occupation	–	6
Total	57	143

Source CDC, Retrieved from http://www.cdc.gov/HAI/organisms/hiv/Surveillance-Occupationally-Acquired-HIV-AIDS.html)

Importantly, some see nPEP and oPEP as essentially the same intervention given they share a theoretical and applied trajectory; therefore, it is not uncommon to find "PEP" used to reference both occupational and nonoccupational exposures. While much is similar between nPEP and oPEP, other than risk context, this context is significant enough that we selected to present them distinctly.

With regard to nPEP, and biomedical interventions in general, two critical, yet distinct, issues evolve that warrants specific consideration: sexual assault and cost-effectiveness. Current postexposure prophylaxis guidelines specify sexual assault as an important use for this preventative treatment. Of concern, the most recent nPEP guidelines note, "documented cases of HIV infection resulting from sexual assault of women or men rarely have been published" (CDC, 2016d, p. 12), yet considerable concern regard accessibility and knowledge of nPEP by the victim and the medical provider attending to the victim (Carrieri et al., 2006; McCausland et al., 2003; Rodriguez et al., 2013). What is critical, and why we raise this issue, is that we must promote as well as make readily available nPEP for all risk exposures to ensure maximized effect given the diversity of behavioral encounters that put a person at risk.

The issue of cost remains an important consideration given ART, on average, costs approximately $2000 per month in 2010 dollars (CDC, 2015b). In 1998, Pinkerton and colleagues conducted a cost-effectiveness analysis of nPEP in association with sexual risk. They concluded "PEP (i.e., nPEP) is highly cost-effective… [yet] should be restricted to partners of infected persons (e.g., sero-discordant couples), to patients reporting unprotected receptive anal intercourse (including condom breakage), and possibly to cases where there is a substantial likelihood that the partner is infected," (p. 1067). The overarching sentiment is that nPEP is a cost-effective prevention tool when targeting high-risk events and when such services are available as well as accessed, which can be more challenging for rural residents who have experienced sexual assault (Annan, 2006; Pinkerton et al., 2004; for additional information see: http://www.aidsmap.com/Cost-effectiveness/page/1746575/).

Pre-exposure Prophylaxis (PrEP)

In 2010, Grant and colleagues published findings from the first PrEP efficacy clinical trial (the iPrEx study). Their theory was that initiating exposure prophylaxis before an exposure can prevent infection while addressing the strict timeframe associated with nPEP; their findings substantiated the theory. There was a 44% reduction in the chance an MSM, their sample population, would acquire HIV when on PrEP. Unlike the recommended three-drug combination for oPEP and nPEP, PrEP is two medications in a single pill (i.e., FTC–TDF; brand name: Truvada®). As mentioned, a significant improvement of PrEP over nPEP is that it eliminates the narrow window (72 h) after an exposure a person must initiate treatment. Although, according to the CDC (2016c):

> PrEP reaches maximum protection from HIV for receptive anal sex at about 7 days of daily use. For all other activities, including insertive anal sex, vaginal sex, and injection drug use, PrEP reaches maximum protection at about 20 days of daily use.

Thus, one must start PrEP at least a week prior to an exposure in order to maximize the protection PrEP offers. Another important consideration regarding PrEP regards adherence—taking the medication as prescribed, i.e., daily. The US Public Health Service's PrEP guidelines (2014) state, "Data from the published studies of daily oral PrEP indicate that medication adherence is critical to achieving the maximum prevention benefit…" (p. 43). In other words, in order to benefit, the person prescribed PrEP needs to take the medication every day. Missing doses can result in reduced effect, meaning PrEP may not prevent infection given the threshold of protection the medication offers is not achieved.

The iPrEx study kicked off a biomedical evolution in HIV prevention; however, this was not the case for several years. Now, 6 years since Grant et al., (2010) published the initial iPrEx findings, and the PrEP evolution is unfolding domestically as well as internationally, a number of populations have the potential to benefit. PrEP is effective in MSM (Buchbinder et al., 2014; Grant et al., 2010, 2014; Molina et al., 2015), heterosexual men and women (Baeten & Celum, 2011; Thigpen et al., 2012; Vann Damme et al., 2012), injection drug users (Choopanya et al., 2013), and transgender women (Buchbinder et al., 2014; Grant et al., 2014). Of these populations, the current U.S. guidelines recommend PrEP for all groups mentioned, except transgender women; PrEP is also not recommended for adolescents, given the lack of data on use among this population at the time of the guidelines issuance, i.e., mid-2014 (US Public Health Service, 2014). PrEP's effectiveness can range from 70% for those who are at risk of HIV from needle sharing to 90% for those engaged in sexual risk taking (CDC, 2016c). Finally, at this time, additional medications are being studied as candidates for PrEP.

Conclusion: Future Direction for HIV Research, Interventions, and Policy

In closing, the CDC reports significant reductions in newly diagnosed HIV cases among nearly all risk groups, yet the number of new diagnoses among gay, bisexual, and other men who have sex with men (MSM), especially, Black/African American and Latino MSM, have increased. To see further reductions in new transmissions, our prevention tool kit must expand in efficacy and coverage—meaning more communities need consistent and affordable access to the interventions that work. The future of primary prevention can significantly benefit from biomedical interventions, specifically TasP, oPEP, nPEP, and PrEP, yet this potential may be truncated by real-world situations that result in non-adherence (see Chan et al., 2016 regarding PrEP nonadherence). In addition, we have yet to understand the consequences of short-term interventions such as oPEP and nPEP on communal level drug resistance—if enough people take nPEP and/or intermittent PrEP, will drug resistance produce a rebound in HIV infection rates; and, what are the longitudinal concerns with antiretroviral use among HIV negative individuals. Further study and education need to be encouraged. In fact, guidelines for optimal care, which should include comprehensive prevention planning, need to be implemented as a standard protocol before initiating any biomedical intervention. Overall, we want to decrease the number of new infections by identifying those infected and making sure they are on TasP while ensuring the uninfected have access to oPEP, nPEP, and PrEP. To do this, we have to eliminate barriers to care, mitigate poverty's impact, repeal criminalization, and eliminate the stigma attached to living with the virus or being at risk for HIV, regardless of where one lives. The future looks bright, but biomedical, behavioral, and structural interventions' potential resides in the availability of resources and leadership to see them applied in all settings.

References

Adimora, A. A., Ramirez, C., Schoenbach, V. J., & Cohen, M. (2014). Policies and politics that promote HIV infection in the southern United States. *AIDS, 28,* 1393–1397.
American Federation for AIDS Research [amfAR]. (2016). Statistics—United States. Retrieved from http://www.amfar.org/about-hiv-and-aids/facts-and-stats/statistics–united-states/

Annan, S. L. (2006). Sexual violence in rural areas: A review of the literature. *Family & Community Health, 29*(3), 164–168.

AVERT. (2016). Treatment as prevention. Retrieved from https://www.avert.org/professionals/hiv-programming/prevention/treatment-as-prevention

Baeten, J., & Celum, C. (2011, July). Antiretroviral pre-exposure prophylaxis for HIV-1 prevention among heterosexual African men and women: The partners PrEP study. In *6th IAS conference on HIV pathogenesis, treatment and prevention* (pp. 17–20). Rome: IAS.

Buchbinder, S. P., Glidden, D. V., Liu, A. Y., McMahan, V., Guanira, J. V., Mayer, K. H., ... & Grant, R. M. (2014). HIV pre-exposure prophylaxis in men who have sex with men and transgender women: A secondary analysis of a phase 3 randomised controlled efficacy trial. *The Lancet Infectious Diseases, 14*(6), 468–475.

Carrieri, M. P., Bendiane, M. K., Moatti, J. P., & Rey, D. (2006). Access to HIV prophylaxis for survivors of sexual assault: The tip of the iceberg (vol. 11, pp. 391, 2006). *Antiviral Therapy, 11*(7), 953–953.

CDC. (1990). Public Health Service statement on management of occupational exposure to human immunodeficiency virus, including considerations regarding zidovudine postexposure use. *MMWR Morbidity and Mortality Weekly Report, 39*(RR01), 1–14.

CDC. (2011). *Surveillance of occupationally acquired HIV/AIDS in healthcare personnel, as of December 2010.* Retrieved from http://www.cdc.gov/HAI/organisms/hiv/Surveillance-Occupationally-Acquired-HIV-AIDS.html

CDC. (2015a). HIV in the Southern United States. Retrieved from http://www.cdc.gov/hiv/pdf/policies/cdc-hiv-in-the-south-issue-brief.pdf

CDC. (2015b). HIV cost effectiveness. Retrieved from http://www.cdc.gov/hiv/programresources/guidance/costeffectiveness/index.html

CDC. (2016a). *Trends in U.S. HIV diagnoses, 2005–2014.* Retrieved from http://www.cdc.gov/nchhstp/newsroom/docs/factsheets/hiv-data-trends-fact-sheet-508.pdf

CDC. (2016b). *Lifetime risk of HIV diagnosis.* Retrieved from http://www.cdc.gov/nchhstp/newsroom/2016/croi-press-release-risk.html

CDC. (2016c). *PrEP.* Retrieved from http://www.cdc.gov/hiv/basics/prep.html

CDC. (2016d). *Updated guidelines for antiretroviral postexposure prophylaxis after sexual, injection drug use, or other nonoccupational exposure to HIV—United States, 2016.* Retrieved from http://www.cdc.gov/hiv/pdf/programresources/cdc-hiv-npep-guidelines.pdf

CDC. (n.d.). *HIV surveillance in urban and nonurban areas through 2013.* Retrieved from www.cdc.gov/hiv/ppt/2013-Urban-Nonurban-slides_508-REV-5.pptx

Centers for Disease Control [CDC]. (1981). Pneumocystis pneumonia — Los Angeles. *Morbidity and Mortality Weekly Report, 30*(21), 1–3. Retrieved from http://www.cdc.gov/mmwr/preview/mmwrhtml/june_5.htm

Chan, P. A., Mena, L., Patel, R., Oldenburg, C. E., Beauchamps, L., Perez-Brumer, A. G., ... & Nunn, A. (2016). Retention in care outcomes for HIV pre-exposure prophylaxis implementation programmes among men who have sex with men in three US cities. *Journal of the International AIDS Society, 19*(1).

Choopanya, K., Martin, M., Suntharasamai, P., Sangkum, U., Mock, P. A., Leethochawalit, M., ... & Chuachoowong, R. (2013). Antiretroviral prophylaxis for HIV infection in injecting drug users in Bangkok, Thailand (the Bangkok Tenofovir Study): A randomised, double-blind, placebo-controlled phase 3 trial. *The Lancet, 381*(9883), 2083–2090.

Cohen, M. S., Chen, Y. Q., McCauley, M., Gamble, T., Hosseinipour, M. C., Kumarasamy, N., ... & Godbole, S. V. (2011). Prevention of HIV-1 infection with early antiretroviral therapy. *New England Journal of Medicine, 365*(6), 493–505.

Cohen, M. S., McCauley, M., & Gamble, T. R. (2012). HIV treatment as prevention and HPTN 052. *Current Opinion in HIV and AIDS, 7*(2), 99.

Connor, E. M., Sperling, R. S., Gelber, R., Kiselev, P., Scott, G., O'Sullivan, M. J., ... & Jimenez, E. (1994). Reduction of maternal-infant transmission of human immunodeficiency virus type 1 with zidovudine treatment. *New England Journal of Medicine, 331*(18), 1173–1180.

Denning, P., & DiNenno, E. (2015). *Communities in crisis: Is there a generalized HIV epidemic in impoverished urban areas of the United States?* Retrieved from http://www.cdc.gov/hiv/group/poverty.html

Fulton County Task Force on HIV/AIDS. (2015). *Phase I progress report: Building the strategy to end AIDS in Fulton County.* Retrieved from http://www.sisterlove.org/wp-content/uploads/2014/10/2015-1201-Strategy-to-End-AIDS-in-Fulton-County-Phase-I.pdf

Georgia Department of Public Health. (n.d. a). *HIV surveillance fact sheet, 2013.* Retrieved from http://dph.georgia.gov/sites/dph.georgia.gov/files/HIV_EPI_Fact_Sheet_Surveillance_2013.pdf

Georgia Department of Public Health. (n.d. b). *HIV surveillance summary, Georgia 2013.* Retrieved from http://dph.georgia.gov/sites/dph.georgia.gov/files/HIV_EPI_2013_Surveillance_Summary.pdf

Gilliam, B. L., Dyer, J. R., Fiscus, S. A., Marcus, C., Zhou, S., Wathen, L., … & Eron Jr, J. J. (1997). Effects of reverse transcriptase inhibitor therapy on the HIV-1 viral burden in semen. *JAIDS Journal of Acquired Immune Deficiency Syndromes, 15*(1), 54–60.

Grant, R. M., Lama, J. R., Anderson, P. L., McMahan, V., Liu, A. Y., Vargas, L., … & Montoya-Herrera, O. (2010). Preexposure chemoprophylaxis for HIV prevention in men who have sex with men. *New England Journal of Medicine, 363*(27), 2587–2599.

Grant, R. M., Anderson, P. L., McMahan, V., Liu, A., Amico, K. R., Mehrotra, M., … & Buchbinder, S. (2014). Uptake of pre-exposure prophylaxis, sexual practices, and HIV incidence in men and transgender women who have sex with men: A cohort study. *The Lancet infectious diseases, 14*(9), 820–829.

Hall, H. I., Li, J., & McKenna, M. T. (2005). HIV in predominantly rural areas of the United States. *The Journal of Rural Health, 21*(3), 245–253.

Heckman, T. G., Somlai, A. M., Peters, J., Walker, J., Otto-Salaj, L., Galdabini, C. A., et al. (1998). Barriers to care among persons living with HIV/AIDS in urban and rural areas. *AIDS Care, 10*(3), 365–375.

Kaplan, J. E., Dominguez, K., Jobarteh, K., & Spira, T. J. (2015). Postexposure prophylaxis against human immunodeficiency virus (HIV): New guidelines from the WHO: A perspective. *Clinical Infectious Diseases, 60*(suppl 3), S196–S199.

Kempf, M. C., McLeod, J., Boehme, A. K., Walcott, M. W., Wright, L., Seal, P., … & Moneyham, L. (2010). A qualitative study of the barriers and facilitators to retention-in-care among HIV-positive women in the rural southeastern United States: Implications for targeted interventions. *AIDS Patient Care and STDs, 24*(8), 515–520.

Kumar, R. S. (2008). Post exposure prophylaxis in HIV. *Oral Hypoglycemic Agents: Where Do We Stand Today? 18*, 752.

Lieb, S., Thompson, D. R., Misra, S., Gates, G. J., Duffus, W. A., Fallon, S. J., … & Southern AIDS Coalition MSM Project Team. (2009). Estimating populations of men who have sex with men in the southern United States. *Journal of Urban Health, 86*(6), 887–901.

McCausland, J. B., Linden, J. A., Degutis, L. C., Ramanujam, P., Sullivan, L. M., & D'Onofrio, G. (2003). Nonoccupational postexposure HIV prevention: Emergency physicians' current practices, attitudes, and beliefs. *Annals of Emergency Eedicine, 42*(5), 651–656.

Molina, J. M., Capitant, C., Spire, B., Pialoux, G., Cotte, L., Charreau, I., … & Raffi, F. (2015). On-demand preexposure prophylaxis in men at high risk for HIV-1 infection. *New England Journal of Medicine, 373*(23), 2237–2246.

Montaner, J. S., Hogg, R., Wood, E., Kerr, T., Tyndall, M., Levy, A. R., et al. (2006). The case for expanding access to highly active antiretroviral therapy to curb the growth of the HIV epidemic. *The Lancet, 368*(9534), 531–536.

National Rural Health Association. (n.d.). *HIV/AIDS in rural America: Disproportionate impact on minority and multicultural populations.* Retrieved fromfile:///C:/Users/necarnes/Downloads/HIVAIDSRuralAmericapolicybriefApril2014%20(2).pdf

O'Malley, J. (2015, April 24). Indiana HIV outbreak, hepatitis C epidemic sparks CDC alert. *The Indianapolis Star.* Retrieved from http://www.indystar.com/story/news/2015/04/24/indiana-hiv-outbreak-hepatitis-epidemic-sparks-cdc-alert/26310539/

Ohl, M. E., & Perencevich, E. (2011). Frequency of human immunodeficiency virus (HIV) testing in urban versus rural areas of the United States: Results from a nationally-representative sample. *BMC Public Health, 11*(1), 1.

Palella, F. J., Delaney, K. M., Moorman, A. C., Loveless, M. O., Fuhrer, J., Satten, G. A., ... & Holmberg, S. D. (1998). HIV Outpatient Study Investigators Declining morbidity and mortality among patients with advanced human immunodeficiency virus infection. *New England Journal of Medicine, 338*(13), 853–860.

Pinkerton, S. D., Holtgrave, D. R., & Bloom, F. R. (1998). Cost-effectiveness of post-exposure prophylaxis following sexual exposure to HIV. *AIDS, 12,* 1067–1078.

Pinkerton, S. D., Martin, J. N., Roland, M. E., Katz, M. H., Coates, T. J., & Kahn, J. O. (2004). Cost-effectiveness of postexposure prophylaxis after sexual or injection-drug exposure to human immunodeficiency virus. *Archives of Internal Medicine, 164*(1), 46–54.

Preston, D. B., D'Augelli, A. R., Kassab, C. D., & Cain, R. E. (2004). The influence of stigma on the sexual risk behavior of rural men who have sex with men. *AIDS Education and Prevention, 16*(4), 291.

Quinn, T. C., Wawer, M. J., Sewankambo, N., Serwadda, D., Li, C., Wabwire-Mangen, F., ... & Gray, R. H. (2000). Viral load and heterosexual transmission of human immunodeficiency virus type 1. *New England Journal of Medicine, 342*(13), 921–929.

Reif, S., Golin, C. E., & Smith, S. R. (2005). Barriers to accessing HIV/AIDS care in North Carolina: Rural and urban differences. *AIDS Care, 17*(5), 558–565.

Reif, S. S., Whetten, K., Wilson, E. R., McAllaster, C., Pence, B. W., Legrand, S., et al. (2014). HIV/AIDS in the Southern USA: A disproportionate epidemic. *AIDS Care, 26*(3), 351–359.

Rodriguez, A., Castel, A. D., Parish, C. L., Willis, S., Feaster, D. J., Kharfen, M., ... & Metsch, L. R. (2013). HIV medical providers' perceptions of the use of antiretroviral therapy as non-occupational post-exposure prophylaxis (nPEP) in two major metropolitan areas. *Journal of Acquired Immune Deficiency Syndromes (1999), 64*(0 1).

Rural Center for AIDS/STD Prevention. (2009). *HIV/AIDS in rural America: Challenges and promising strategies.* Retrieved from http://www.indiana.edu/~aids/factsheets/factsheet23.pdf

Schreiner, M. C., Stingl, G., Rieger, A., & Jalili, A. (2013). P4. 049 lopinavir/ritonavir in combination with tenofovir/emtricitabine as post exposure prophylaxis (PEP) to HIV-an effective and well tolerated regimen. *Sexually Transmitted Infections, 89*(Suppl 1), A303–A304.

Sowell, R. L., Lowenstein, A., Moneyham, L., Demi, A., Mizuno, Y., & Seals, B. F. (1997). Resources, stigma, and patterns of disclosure in rural women with HIV infection. *Public Health Nursing, 14*(5), 302–312.

Sutton, M., Anthony, M. N., Vila, C., McLellan-Lemal, E., & Weidle, P. J. (2010). HIV testing and HIV/AIDS treatment services in rural counties in 10 southern states: Service provider perspectives. *The Journal of Rural Health, 26*(3), 240–247.

Thigpen, M. C., Kebaabetswe, P. M., Paxton, L. A., Smith, D. K., Rose, C. E., Segolodi, T. M., ... & Mutanhaurwa, R. (2012). Antiretroviral preexposure prophylaxis for heterosexual HIV transmission in Botswana. *New England Journal of Medicine, 367*(5), 423–434.

U.S. Department of Agriculture. (2015). *Rural poverty and well-being.* Retrieved from http://www.ers.usda.gov/topics/rural-economy-population/rural-poverty-well-being/geography-of-poverty.aspx

U.S. Public Health Service. (2014). *Preexposure Prophylaxis for the prevention of HIV infection in the United States—2014 clinical practice guideline.* Retrieved from http://www.cdc.gov/hiv/pdf/prepguidelines2014.pdf

Van Damme, L., Corneli, A., Ahmed, K., Agot, K., Lombaard, J., Kapiga, S., ... & Temu, L. (2012). Preexposure prophylaxis for HIV infection among African women. *New England Journal of Medicine, 367*(5), 411–422.

Vyavaharkar, M., Glover, S., Leonhirth, D., & Probst, J. (2013). *HIV/AIDS in rural America: Prevalence and service availability.* Retrieved from http://rhr.sph.sc.edu/report/%2811-1%29HIV%20AIDS%20in%20Rural%20America.pdf

World Health Organization [WHO]. (n.d.). *Global health observatory (GHO) data—HIV/AIDS.* Retrieved from http://www.who.int/gho/hiv/en/

Yannessa, J. F., Reece, M., & Basta, T. B. (2008). HIV provider perspectives: The impact of stigma on substance abusers living with HIV in a rural area of the United States. *AIDS Patient Care and STDs, 22*(8), 669–675.

Chapter 6
Pediatric/Adolescent HIV: Legal and Ethical Issues

Tiffany Chenneville

Introduction

Health professionals, including mental health professionals and others working with children and adolescents with HIV, are likely to encounter a variety of situations requiring familiarity with law and ethical practices. The purpose of this chapter is to describe important legal and ethical considerations when working with children and adolescents with HIV. While these considerations are important in all settings, they may be particularly relevant in rural settings where resources are limited and health disparities are prevalent.

Legal Considerations for Pediatric/Adolescent HIV Treatment and Research

Healthcare practitioners, educators, and others working with children and adolescents with HIV or those at risk for contracting HIV should take into consideration federal and state laws that may affect their activities. Familiarity with these laws is particularly important when working in rural settings. While some research suggests HIV-related stigma is similar in urban and rural settings (French, Greeff, Watson, & Doak, 2015), there is at least some evidence to suggest stigma is higher in rural settings (Bunn, Solomon, Varni, Miller, Forehand, & Ashikaga, 2008; Costelloe et al., 2015).

T. Chenneville (✉)
Department of Psychology, University of South Florida
St. Petersburg, 140 USFSP Harborwalk Avenue South, DAV 117,
St. Petersburg, FL 33701, USA
e-mail: chennevi@mail.usf.edu

© Springer International Publishing AG 2017
F.M. Parks et al. (eds.), *HIV/AIDS in Rural Communities*,
DOI 10.1007/978-3-319-56239-1_6

Federal Laws

There are several federal laws that protect the rights of children and adolescents with HIV. Among these are the Health Information and Portability Accountability Act (HIPAA, 1996), the Americans with Disabilities Act and its amendments (ADA, 1990a; ADA Amendments Act, 2008), the Rehabilitation Act of 1973 (1973), the Individuals with Disabilities Education Act (IDEA, 1990, 2004), and the Federal Educational Rights and Privacy Act (FERPA, 1974). Each of these laws and their applicability to children and adolescents with HIV is described in the paragraphs to follow.

HIPAA. HIPAA (1996) protects confidential health information. In the case of HIV, protected health information (PHI) includes disease status to include not only HIV, but also any other disease associated with HIV as well as information about HIV-related medical exams or tests. Exposure to HIV also is considered PHI. HIPAA protection is important for respecting human dignity and preventing the misuse of data and/or discrimination against people with health conditions such as HIV (Bădărău, 2013). The release of confidential health information—intentionally or unintentionally—may result in fines or incarceration. While HIPAA is probably most relevant to health practitioners working with children and adolescents with HIV in treatment settings, it also has relevance to researchers as well as educators given that HIPAA laws extend to public schools, colleges, and universities (see Chenneville, 2014 for a complete description of the applicability of HIPAA as it relates to HIV in school settings). Under HIPAA laws, parents have the right to access their children's medical information and to ensure that erroneous information is corrected.

HIPAA does allow for disclosure of PHI under certain conditions (Bădărău, 2013). Generally speaking, PHI can be disclosed for treatment purposes, for obtaining payment, for healthcare operations, or when there is a valid authorization. Other exceptions also can be made. For example, PHI including HIV status may be released for victims of violence, for whistleblowers, and for activities related to public health oversight. Further, disclosure may be mandated in response to court orders or subpoenas. Some institutional review boards (IRBs) also will provide waivers to researchers so that PHI can be used within the context of research. These exceptions are highly relevant to work with children and adolescents with HIV and/or at risk for contracting HIV. For example, HIV researchers often must have access to PHI in order to complete their studies and also for the protection of their participants, for example, when a participant with HIV living in a state with active HIV criminalization laws reveals that s/he is having, or has had, sex with someone who is unaware of his/her HIV status. More information about HIV criminalization laws is included below.

ADA. The ADA (1990a) is a civil rights law that protects people with disabilities by making discrimination against a person with a disability unlawful. Under the

ADA, disability is defined as a "physical or mental impairment that substantially limits one or more major life activities" (ADA, 1990b, p. 328). The ADA applies to nearly all entities including schools. Although there are some questions about whether or not HIV and AIDS are disabling per se (Larson, 2015), it is generally understood that discriminating against people with HIV or AIDS is illegal under the ADA. This means it is unlawful for employers to discriminate against people, including children and adolescents, with HIV. This also means it is unlawful for health providers to refuse to treat children and adolescents with HIV on the basis of their disease, or for educators to discriminate against children and adolescents with HIV who are students in a school setting. This law is extremely important given documented evidence of discrimination against people living with HIV (e.g., Gagnon, 2015; Graham, 2014), particularly in rural settings.

Rehabilitation Act of 1973. Similar to the ADA, Section 504 of the Rehabilitation Act of 1973 is a civil rights law that prohibits discrimination based on disability. However, unlike the ADA, which applies to nearly all entities, Section 504 of the Rehabilitation Act applies only to entities receiving federal funds. This includes schools and is, therefore, an important law for students with HIV. Because a free and appropriate education must be afforded to all children and adolescents, adequate accommodations must be granted to students with HIV to ensure they have equal access to education. This means that students with HIV may be afforded educational modifications in the regular classroom setting. Unfortunately, many families do not have access to these accommodations because they do not disclose their child's HIV status to school personnel due to fears of HIV-related stigma. This may be particularly prevalent in rural settings where families fear that disclosure of HIV status to the school may result in unintended disclosure to the community.

FERPA. FERPA, also known as the Buckley Amendment, safeguards the privacy of school records. Under FERPA, only individuals with a legitimate need to know should be granted access to confidential school records. For students with HIV, this is extremely important. However, perceptions vary with regard to who in a school setting has a legitimate need to know a child's HIV status. In an empirical study of elementary school principal's decisions about disclosure of confidential medical information in the school setting, Chenneville (2008) found that disclosure decisions varied significantly based on the child's diagnosis and the presence of symptomatology. The focus in schools should be the use of universal precautions, not disclosure of HIV status to teachers and staff. After all, there will be students who do not even know they are infected with HIV. Thus, if the goal of disclosure is transmission prevention, the only way to assure this is through the use of universal precautions. This is true not only for HIV but also other communicable diseases. Beyond fear of transmission, some may believe teachers need to know HIV status in order to best serve the student. However, it is important to weigh the potential benefits of such disclosure against the potential risks especially in light of existing HIV-related stigma and discrimination, particularly in rural settings.

IDEA. IDEA is a federal law that further ensures students with disabilities are afforded a free and appropriate education. Exceptional student education (ESE) programs are a function of IDEA. While there is not an ESE classification for students with HIV, they may qualify for ESE services under the Other Health Impaired, or similar, category. Alternatively, because of the neurodevelopmental implications of HIV, students with HIV may qualify for ESE services because of a learning or behavioral disorder regardless of whether their HIV status is known. For a comprehensive description of developmental issues among children and adolescents with HIV, see Nichols (2017).

State Laws

There is wide variation in state laws affecting HIV testing, treatment, and prevention. Health providers, educators, and others working with children and adolescents should familiarize themselves with HIV-related laws in their state, particularly those related to HIV testing, HIV criminalization, and sexuality education. In the sections to follow, HIV-related state laws are described. However, because laws are continuously changing, readers are referred to the Centers for Disease Control and Prevention website at http://www.cdc.gov/hiv/policies/law/states/ or the Center for HIV Law and Policy website at http://www.hivlawandpolicy.org/state-hiv-laws for up-to-date information about relevant HIV laws in their state.

HIV Testing Laws. Most states allow adolescent minors access to reproductive health care without parental permission under minor consent statutes (English, 2007; English, Bass, Boyle, & Eshragh, 2010). These laws allow minors to provide their own consent to confidential treatment and, in some states, include provisions for financial support to help cover medical costs. Minor consent laws related to HIV vary with some states allowing adolescents to consent to HIV testing, but not treatment if they test positive. Thus, it is very important for health providers including HIV testing counselors to understand the laws in their state. HIV researchers also should be familiar with their state's laws. Providing Institutional Review Boards (IRBs) with information about minor consent laws related to HIV testing and treatment can be helpful when seeking waivers of parental permission for participation in research, which often are important to ensure IRBs do not act as barriers for much needed HIV research among youth (Mustanski & Fisher, 2016). Of note, most minor consent laws do not allow minors to consent to HIV prevention services (Moore, Paul, McGuire, & Majumder, 2016), which may affect both healthcare delivery and research.

HIV Criminalization Laws. HIV criminalization laws make it illegal for someone with HIV to have sexual relations with someone who does not know their

HIV status. Such laws are the source of much controversy with many arguing that criminalizing HIV undermines public health efforts related to HIV prevention (Burris, Beletsky, Burleson, Case, & Lazzarini, 2007; Galletly & Pinkerton, 2004, 2006; Galletly & Dickson-Gomez, 2009; O'Byrne, 2012). HIV advocacy and other professional groups are calling for an end to HIV criminalization on the grounds that these laws are unethical and violate human rights. Examples include the Center for HIV Law and Policy (2010) and the HIV Medicine Association (2012). In addition, the American Psychological Association (2016) recently passed a resolution opposing HIV criminalization. Nonetheless, HIV criminalization laws currently exist in nearly half of all states in the US, many of which make it a felony not to disclose HIV status to a sexual partner and some of which require that those convicted be included on the sex offenders registry (Galletly, DiFranceisco, & Pinkerton, 2009). Adolescents are not immune to such laws. Therefore, it is vital that health professionals and others working with youth with HIV be aware of whether or not HIV criminalization laws exist in their state. Researchers working in states with HIV criminalization laws are encouraged to obtain a certificate of confidentiality from their IRB to protect participants. To obtain up-to-date information about HIV criminalization laws by state, please refer to the Center for HIV Law and Policy website at http://www.hivlawandpolicy.org/state-hiv-laws.

Sexuality Education Laws. Sex education for children and adolescents enrolled in public schools is governed by states. For years, federal funding for state-administered sexuality education was tied to the use of abstinence-only curricula through legislation such as the 1996 Welfare Reform Act, which authorized the release of $50 million over five years to states agreeing to promote the abstinence-until-marriage message in their sexuality curricula. Recognizing the importance of comprehensive sexuality education, the Obama Administration attempted to cut funding for abstinence-only programs. However, abstinence-only supporters continue to fight for funding.

Currently, sex education in public schools is mandated in 24 states while HIV instruction is mandated in 33 states and the District of Columbia (National Conference of State Legislatures, 2016). In 20 states offering HIV or sex education, there is a requirement that such education be "medically, factually, or technically accurate" (National Conference of State Legislatures, 2016) although how states determine the accuracy of the education being provided varies. Parental involvement in sexuality education programs is permitted in 38 states, and parents can opt out of sexuality education for their children in 35 states. Only four states require parental consent for sexuality education. It is important for HIV educators, in particular, to be familiar with their state's laws surrounding sexuality education. For more information about state sex and HIV education policies, please refer to the Henry J. Kaiser Family Foundation website at http://kff.org/hivaids/state-indicator/sexhiv-education-policy/.

Ethical Considerations for Pediatric/Adolescent HIV Treatment and Research

Most health professions are guided by some variation of the following ethical principles: beneficence/nonmaleficence, integrity, fidelity, responsibility, justice, and respect for personal rights and dignity. Because these principles are intertwined in many ways, their application often results in ethical conflicts. The ethical issues most commonly encountered by professionals working in the area of pediatric/adolescent HIV surround confidentiality, disclosure, informed consent, and cultural competence. These issues are summarized in the sections to follow.

Confidentiality

Confidentiality is the means by which an individual's privacy is protected. While privacy is a personal right that is focused on the individual, confidentiality is a professional duty that is focused on information (Nagy, 2011). Patients and research participants have come to expect confidentiality of personal information and records. It is well understood that HIV disease status and its correlates constitute protected health information that should remain confidential. However, complications can arise when working with children and adolescents with HIV. The question becomes who owns the right to privacy—the child/minor adolescent or the parent? While less of an issue when working with younger children, this situation presents a relatively common issue when working with adolescents who may, for a variety of reasons, wish to withhold from their parents information about their health. This is particularly true when working with adolescents with HIV or at risk for HIV who do not want their parents to have access to information about their sexual health. In these situations, practitioners and researchers are put in the uncomfortable position of balancing the adolescent's right to privacy with the parents' right to information within the context of law and ethics surrounding confidentiality.

Based on standards of clinical practice and available research and taking into consideration both law and ethics, the Society for Adolescent Medicine (SAM) advocates for confidential health care for adolescents (Ford, English, & Sigman, 2004). SAM's position is based on the belief that protecting the confidence of adolescent health records is consistent with the maturity level and autonomy rights of adolescents and that, without such protection, adolescents may not gain access to the health care they need. SAM supports fostering effective communication between parents and adolescents and believes parental involvement should be encouraged but not mandated. SAM's position applies to research as well as clinical care. SAM's position statement provides a good model for thinking about how to approach confidentiality issues when working with adolescents with HIV.

A situation that sometimes arises for health professionals, including mental health professionals, working with adolescents with HIV is what to do when the adolescent shares that s/he is engaging in sexual relations with someone who is unaware of his/her HIV status. This invokes a dilemma because health professionals have an ethical and legal duty to maintain confidentiality but also have an ethical and legal duty to protect others from harm. The confidentiality versus duty to protect dilemma was highlighted in a landmark court case, Tarasoff v. Regents of the University of California (1974, 1976), where a psychologist failed to warn a third party of potential harm. This case went all the way to the Supreme Court where a ruling was made that mental health professionals have a duty to protect third parties where there is a known threat. The applicability of the Tarasoff ruling to cases involving HIV is controversial. Legal impact aside, the ethical dilemma persists for health professionals. On the continuum of confidentiality to disclosure, medical professionals who typically adhere to a public health model may lean more toward limited disclosure of HIV status. This typically takes the form of compliance with partner notification programs administered through local health departments. Mental health professionals, on the other hand, whose rapport with clients relies so heavily on trust within the therapeutic relationship, are more likely to err in favor of maintaining complete confidentiality while working with the client to overcome barriers to disclosure. For example, the American Psychological Association (1991) advocates for strict confidentiality, resolving that a duty to protect from HIV infection should not be imposed on psychologists.

Disclosure

Health professionals and others working with children and adolescents with HIV likely will confront issues regarding disclosure, either disclosure to the child about his/her own HIV status in the case of children perinatally infected or the child/adolescent's disclosure of their HIV status to others. The latter applies to children perinatally or behaviorally infected. For a variety of reasons, parents often struggle with disclosing to their child that s/he has HIV and, in fact, most do not disclose until adolescence (Sahay, 2013). In some cases, the mother or both parents also have HIV, which means disclosure to the child will require self-disclosure which, in turn, may require the sharing of information about behaviors associated with the parent's acquisition of HIV (e.g., drug use, sexual behavior). In cases of adoption, disclosure of HIV status to the child may also require disclosure of adoption status and/or disclosure of information about biological parental death due to AIDS. Maternal guilt and fear of the child's reaction serve as barriers to disclosure. In addition, parents often fear that their family's HIV status will be shared with others (e.g., school, community, extended family members) once the child knows. This fear may be compounded in rural settings where, as described above, there is at least some evidence to suggest HIV-related stigma may be higher. Nonetheless, disclosure is important. The American Academy of Pediatrics Committee on Pediatric AIDS (1999) issued a statement in support of disclosure of HIV status to adolescents if not younger children.

Disclosing HIV status to sexual partners is important for preventing the transmission of HIV to others. Research has demonstrated that sexual partners are more likely to consistently use safer sex practices when both are aware that one has HIV (Dempsey, MacDonell, Naar-King, Lau, & Adolescent Medicine Trials Network for HIV/ AIDS Interventions, 2012). Yet, for a variety of reasons, youth do not always disclose to their sexual partners that they are living with HIV (Dempsey et al., 2012; Marhefka, Valentin, Pinto, Demetriou, Wiznia, & Mellins, 2011; Chenneville, Lynn, Peacock, Turner, & Marhefka, 2014). Additionally, there is some evidence to suggest that disclosure concerns are greater in rural settings (Costelloe et al., 2015). Some of the reasons for nondisclosure include worries that the sexual partner will not understand, will not want to be with them anymore, or will tell others (Chenneville et al., 2014). Youth also have cited insufficient skills (i.e., not knowing how to disclose) as a reason for nondisclosure to sexual partners. Unfortunately, failure to disclose HIV status to sexual partners not only increases the risk of HIV transmission to others, but also may result in legal consequences for the adolescent, as in the case of HIV criminalization laws, or the healthcare professionals treating them, as in the case of the application of the Tarasoff duty to protect. For a more comprehensive review of issues related to disclosure, please refer to Marhefka, Turner, and Chenneville (2017).

Informed Consent

At the crux of ethical concerns about adolescent HIV treatment and research is the issue of informed consent, which is crucial for respecting individual autonomy as reflected in the Nuremberg Code (National Institutes of Health, 1949), the Declaration of Helsinki (World Medical Association, 2004), and the Belmont Report (National Commission for the Protection of Human Subjects of Biomedical and Behavioral Research, 1979). Federal Policy for the Protection of Human Subjects, also known as the Common Rule, outlines the requirement for informed consent from all research participants unless waived in accordance with regulations by an IRB (Public Welfare General Requirements for Informed Consent, 2003). In the case of minors who, because of their age, are unable to provide informed consent, parental permission and child assent is required except under special situations (e.g., when a child has been emancipated from his/her parents or legal guardians). Child assent refers to a minor's affirmative agreement to participate in research and typically is required for children age seven and older. Mere failure to object is not enough to qualify as assent. Assent from minors is increasingly valued in treatment settings as well. Informed consent and assent involve several elements. In addition to full disclosure on the part of the clinician/researcher and voluntary agreement on the part of the patient/client/research participant, informed consent assumes the person providing consent truly comprehends the information presented. This can be an issue when working with minors, particularly adolescents. As described above when discussing minor consent laws, there may be situations where adolescents' access to medical care is dependent on their ability to consent for themselves. In such situations, health professionals, researchers, and others working with adolescents with HIV must balance protection with respect for autonomy (Chenneville, Sibille, & Bendell-Estroff, 2010). Concerns about minor consent notwithstanding, over protection will diminish autonomy, which can have deleterious effects. Not only may overly stringent consent laws impede treatment for adolescents with HIV, but adolescent HIV research is negatively affected by legal and ethical positions that are overly paternal. For example, Mustanski and Fisher (2016) report that HIV rates are increasing among teens who identify as gay or bisexual as a result of IRB barriers to research. For a more comprehensive review of issues related to informed consent, please refer to Fisher, Arbeit, and Chenneville (2017).

Cultural Competence

Ethical practice and cultural competence are inextricably linked. Fisher (2014) describes ethical contextualism as the practice of considering a client's context to include cultural values and lived experience within the broader context of the health professional's own moral values. Although definitions of cultural competence vary, the principles of cultural competence involve respecting cultural differences and acknowledging that culture is important as well as attempting to minimize any negative consequences resulting from cultural differences (Paasche-Orlow, 2004). Because health disparities related to HIV are well documented (Aral, Adimora, & Fenton, 2008; Chu & Selwyn, 2008), the importance of cultural competence for decreasing healthcare disparities (Betancourt, Green, Carrillo, & Park, 2005) and delivering evidence-based interventions (Engebretson, Mahoney, & Carlson, 2008) cannot be ignored. Indeed, many health organizations have published standards and position statements promoting cultural competence (e.g., American Medical Association, American Psychological Association, and American Nurses Association). Health professionals and others working with children and adolescents with HIV should familiarize themselves with interventions designed to improve cultural competence as a means to decrease health disparities. As an example, the American Academy of Nursing recommends strategies for decreasing health disparities by increasing cultural competence through education, practice, research, policy, and advocacy (Giger, Davidhizar, Purnell, Harden, Phillips, & Strickland, 2007).

Cultural competence is of particular importance in rural settings where risk behaviors related to HIV are prevalent and include early onset of sexual activity and substance use. Further, in rural settings, the stigmatization of people with HIV and key populations at risk for HIV (e.g., racial and sexual minorities) is high and often intersects with disparate levels of poverty and strongly held religious/spiritual beliefs. These factors combined make the design and implementation of HIV prevention and intervention programs in rural settings both financially and practically difficult. Involving families in efforts to decrease risk behaviors associated with HIV among youth may be critical. For example, in a randomized controlled trial, the Strong African American Families Program demonstrated success for altering parenting practices to those shown to serve a protective role in risk behaviors associated with HIV among youth (Murry, Berkel, Chen, Brody, Gibbons, & Gerrard, 2011).

Foster (2007) provides a framework for HIV prevention in rural communities where stigma, fear, and denial contribute significantly to existing health disparities. This framework addresses stigma, fear, and denial through a "prevention engine" that eliminates barriers that include misinformation, myths, and distrust of HIV initiatives through education and training focused on community empowerment, cultural competence skill development, and social action. While this framework originally was designed to address African American communities, it can be applied to other marginalized communities as well to include other racial minorities, sexual minorities, and impoverished communities where stigma, fear, and denial contribute to health disparities.

Legal and Ethical Decision-Making Related to Pediatric/Adolescent HIV Treatment and Research

Because legal and ethical issues related to HIV treatment and research for children and adolescents are so intertwined, decision-making should involve a consideration of both law and ethics as well as developmental and family factors. Fisher (2017) proposes a goodness-of-fit ethical framework (GFE), which draws on relational ethics (Fisher, 1999, 2000). Relational ethics combine aspects of Kohlberg's (1984) justice-based approach, which focuses on respect, beneficence, and fairness with Gilligan's (1982) care-based approach, which focuses on interpersonal context. Historically applied primarily to ethical issues related to research, recently GFE has been applied to clinical practice as well. GFE focuses on the importance of designing procedures that provide a good "fit" between the characteristics of the child/adolescent (e.g., cognitive and emotional maturity), the family system, and the unique demands of the research or clinical context (Masty & Fisher, 2008). GFE has been applied in a variety of health contexts, to include HIV, and is highly valued as an evidenced-based approach to ethics. The GFE framework may be particularly relevant in rural settings given its emphasis on context. For example, HIV stigma and limited resources are important contextual factors that need to be considered when developing HIV research protocols and treatment interventions that reflect a good fit between the child, the family, and the context in rural settings.

Also, as described above, ethical contextualism or the practice of considering a client's context to include cultural values and lived experience within the broader context of the health professional's own moral values is important (Fisher, 2014). In rural settings in particular, there may be differences between the health professional, the minor client, and the family with regard to moral values, cultural values, and lived experience.

Other models, which are more situation specific, do exist. For example, Chenneville, Sibille, and Bendell-Estroff (2010) proposed a model for balancing autonomy rights with the need for protection when working with minor children and adolescents with HIV. This model acknowledges that over protection may impede the rights of children and adolescents and highlights the importance of decisional capacity as an important construct when confronted with ethical decisions surrounding consent and assent. This model draws on existing work in the area of decisional capacity (Grisso & Appelbaum, 1998a, b; Grisso, Appelbaum, & Hill-Fotouhi, 1997), which involves four components: understanding, appreciation, reasoning, and ability to express a choice. Chenneville, Sibille, and Bendell-Estroff (2010) advocate for the assessment of decisional capacity of minor children and adolescents with HIV as a means by which to balance the extremes of the protection-autonomy continuum (see Fig. 6.1). Chenneville (2000) also proposed a model for approaching the confidentiality versus duty to protect dilemma described above. This model involves a step-wise action plan for health professionals that takes into consideration both law and ethics (see Fig. 6.2). See Chenneville (2000) for an example of the application of this model, which has relevance to rural settings.

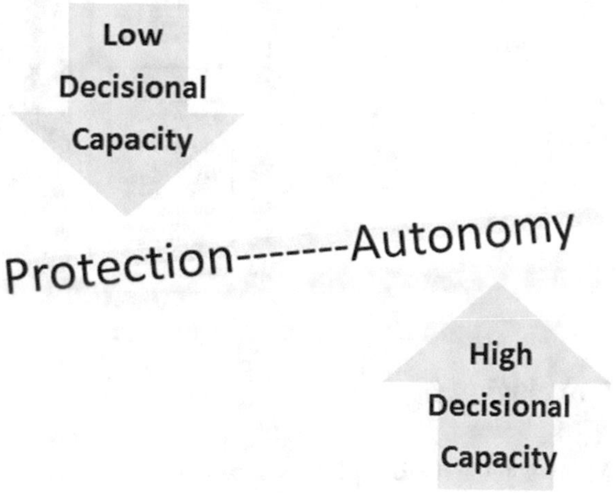

Fig. 6.1 A model for balancing autonomy rights with the need for protection for children with HIV (see Chenneville et al. 2010)

Low
Decisional
Capacity

Protection-------Autonomy

High
Decisional
Capacity

Fig. 6.2 Model for
approaching the
confidentiality versus duty to
protect dilemma when
treating clients with HIV
(see Chenneville 2000)

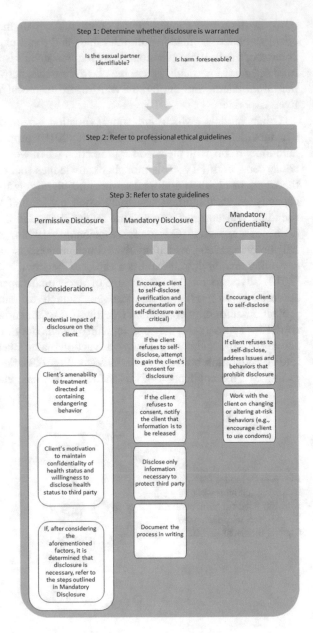

Conclusion

Many legal and ethical issues surround pediatric and adolescent HIV treatment and
research. It is important for health professionals and others working with children
and adolescents with HIV to be aware of the variety of ethical and legal issues they

are likely to encounter as described in this chapter. Health professionals also are well advised to familiarize themselves with the ethical frameworks and decision-making models that will assist them with addressing the legal and ethical dilemmas they encounter. This is particularly true in rural settings where health disparities are high and resources often are limited. Health professionals, researchers, policy makers, and advocates are encouraged to work together to ensure that existing laws and ethical practices work for and not against the youth they serve.

Acknowledgements   I would like to thank Hunter Drake for his contributions to this chapter.

References

ADA Amendments Act of 2008 (ADAAA). (2008). P.L. no. 110–325, 122 STAT. 3553.

American Academy of Pediatrics Committee on Pediatric AIDS. (1999). Disclosure of illness status to children and adolescents with HIV infection. *Pediatrics, 103*(1), 164–166.

American Psychological Association. (1991). Legal liability related to confidentiality and the prevention of HIV transmission. Retrieved from http://www.apa.org/about/policy/confidentiality.aspx

American Psychological Association. (2016). Resolution opposing HIV criminalization. Retrieved from http://www.apa.org/about/policy/hiv-criminalization.aspx

Americans with Disabilities Act of 1990 (ADA). (1990a). P.L. no. 101–336, 42 USC Section 12101 *et seq.*

Americans with Disabilities Act of 1990. (1990b). P.L. no. 101–336, Section 1, 104 Stat. 328.

Aral, S. O., Adimora, A. A., & Fenton, K. A. (2008). Understanding and responding to disparities in HIV and other sexually transmitted infections in African Americans. *The Lancet, 372*(9635), 337–340. doi:10.1016/S0140-6736(08)61118-6

Bădărău, D. O. (2013). Disclosure laws. In *Mental health practitioner's guide to HIV/AIDS* (pp. 197–200). New York: Springer. doi:10.1007/978-1-4614-5283-6_34

Betancourt, J. R., Green, A. R., Carrillo, J. E., & Park, E. R. (2005). Cultural competence and health care disparities: Key perspectives and trends. *Health Affairs, 24*(2), 499–505. doi:10.1377/hlthaff.24.2.499

Bunn, J. Y., Solomon, S. E., Varni, S. E., Miller, C. T., Forehand, R. L., & Ashikaga, T. (2008). Urban-rural differences in motivation to control prejudice toward people with HIV/AIDS: The impact of perceived identifiability in the community. *The Journal of Rural Health, 24*(3), 285–291. doi:10.1111/j.1748-0361.2008.00170.x

Burris, S., Beletsky, L., Burleson, J. A., Case, P., & Lazzarini, Z. (2007). Do criminal laws influence HIV risk behavior? An empirical trial. *Arizona State Law Journal.* doi:10.2139/ssrn.913323, doi:10.2139/ssrn.913323

Center for HIV Law and Policy. (2010). Ending and defending against HIV criminalization: State and federal laws and prosecutions. Available at http://www.Hivlawandpolicy.org/resources/ending-and-defending-against-hiv-criminalization-state-and-federal-laws-and-prosecutions

Chenneville, T. (2000). HIV, confidentiality, and duty to protect: A decision-making model. *Professional Psychology: Research and Practice, 31*(6), 661–670. doi:10.1037//0735-7028.31.6.661

Chenneville, T. (2008). Results from an empirical study of school principals' decisions about disclosure of HIV status. *Journal of HIV/AIDS Prevention & Education for Adolescents & Children, 8*(2), 9–30. doi:10.1300/j499v08n02_02

Chenneville, T. (2014). Best practices in responding to HIV in the school setting. In A. Thomas & P. Harrison (Eds.), *Best practices in school psychology* (6th ed., pp. 1389–1402). Bethesda, MD: National Association of School Psychologists.

Chenneville, T., Lynn, V., Peacock, B., Turner, D., & Marhefka, S. (2014). Disclosure of HIV status among female youth with HIV. *Ethics and Behavior, 25*(4), 314–331. doi:10.1080/10508422.2014.934371

Chenneville, T., Sibille, K., & Bendell-Estroff, D. (2010). Decisional capacity among minors with HIV: A model for balancing autonomy rights with the need for protection. *Ethics and Behavior, 20*(2), 83–94. doi:10.1080/10508421003595901

Chu, C., & Selwyn, P. A. (2008). Current health disparities in HIV/AIDS. *The AIDS Reader, 18*(3), 144–144.

Costelloe, S., Kemppainen, J., Brion, J., MacKain, S., Reid, P., Frampton, A., & Rigsbee, E. (2015). Impact of anxiety and depressive symptoms on perceptions of stigma in persons living with HIV disease in rural versus urban North Carolina. *AIDS Care, 27*(12), 1425–1428. doi:10.1080/09540121.2015.1114993

Dempsey, A. G., MacDonell, K. E., Naar-King, S., Lau, C. Y., & Adolescent Medicine Trials Network for HIV/AIDS Interventions. (2012). Patterns of disclosure among youth who are HIV-positive: A multisite study. *Journal of Adolescent Health, 50*, 315–317. doi:10.1016/j.jadohealth.2011.06.003

Engebretson, J., Mahoney, J., & Carlson, E. D. (2008). Cultural competence in the era of evidence-based practice. *Journal of Professional Nursing, 24*(3), 172–178. doi:10.1016/j.profnurs.2007.10.012

English, A. (2007). Sexual and reproductive health care for adolescents: Legal rights and policy challenges. *Adolescent Medicine: State of the Art Reviews, 18*(3), 571–581.

English, A., Bass, L., Boyle, A. D., & Eshragh, F. (2010). *State minor consent laws: A summary* (3rd ed.). Chapel Hill, North Carolina: Center for Adolescent Health & the Law.

Family Educational Rights and Privacy Act of 1974 (FERPA). (1974). 20 USC Section 1232g.

Fisher, C. B. (1999). *Relational ethics and research with vulnerable populations.* In *Reports on research involving persons with mental disorders that may affect decision-making capacity* (Vol. 2, pp. 29–49). Commissioned Papers by the National Bioethics Advisory Commission. Rockville, MD: National Bioethics Advisory Commission. Retrieved August 1, 2015, from http://www.bioethics.gov/reports/past_commissions/nbac_mental2.pdf

Fisher, C. B. (2000). Relational ethics in psychological research: One feminist's journey. In M. M. Brabeck (Ed.), *Practicing feminist ethics in psychology: Psychology of women book series* (pp. 125–142). Washington, DC, US: American Psychological Association. doi:10.1037/10343-006

Fisher, C. B. (2014). Multicultural ethics in professional psychology practice, consulting, and training. In F. T. Leong (Ed.), *APA handbook of multicultural psychology, Vol. 2: Applications and training* (pp. 35–57). American Psychological Association: Washington, DC. doi:10.1037/14187-003

Fisher, C. B. (2017). *Decoding the ethics code: A practical guide for psychologists* (4th ed.). Los Angeles, CA: Sage Publications.

Fisher, C. B., Arbeit, M., & Chenneville, T. (2017). Goodness-of-fit ethics for practice and research involving children and adolescents with HIV. In T. Chenneville (Ed.), *A clinical guide to pediatric HIV: Bridging the gaps between research and practice*. New York: Springer.

Ford, C., English, A., & Sigman, G. (2004). Confidential health care for adolescents: Position paper of the society for adolescent medicine. *Journal of Adolescent Health, 35*(2), 160–167. doi:10.1016/S1054-139X(04)00086-2

Foster, P. H. (2007). Use of stigma, fear, and denial in development of a framework for prevention of HIV/AIDS in rural African American communities. *Family & Community Health, 30*(4), 318–327.

French, H., Greeff, M., Watson, M. J., & Doak, C. M. (2015). HIV stigma and disclosure experiences of people living with HIV in an urban and a rural setting. *AIDS Care, 27*(8), 1042–1046. doi:10.1080/09540121.2015.1020747

Gagnon, M. (2015). Feature: Re-thinking HIV-related stigma in health care settings: A qualitative study. *Journal of the Association of Nurses in AIDS Care, 26*, 703–719. doi:10.1016/j.jana. 2015.07.005

Galletly, C. L., & Dickson-Gomez, J. (2009). HIV seropositive status disclosure to prospective sex partners and criminal laws that require it: Perspectives of persons living with HIV. *International Journal of STD & AIDS, 20*(9), 613–618. doi:10.1258/ijsa.2008.008417

Galletly, C. L., DiFranceisco, W., & Pinkerton, S. D. (2009). HIV-positive persons' awareness and understanding of their state's criminal HIV disclosure law. *AIDS and Behavior, 13*(6), 1262–1269. doi:10.1007/s10461-008-9477-y

Galletly, C. L., & Pinkerton, S. D. (2004). Toward rational criminal HIV exposure laws. *The Journal of Law, Medicine & Ethics, 32*(2), 327–337. doi:10.1111/j.1748-720x.2004.tb00479.x

Galletly, C. L., & Pinkerton, S. D. (2006). Conflicting messages: How criminal HIV disclosure laws undermine public health efforts to control the spread of HIV. *AIDS and Behavior, 10*(5), 451–461. doi:10.1007/s10461-006-9117-3

Giger, J., Davidhizar, R. E., Purnell, L., Harden, J. T., Phillips, J., & Strickland, O. (2007). American academy of nursing expert panel report developing cultural competence to eliminate health disparities in ethnic minorities and other vulnerable populations. *Journal of Transcultural Nursing, 18*(2), 95–102. doi:10.1177/1043659606298618

Gilligan, C. (1982). *In a different voice*. Cambridge, MA: Harvard University Press.

Graham, J. M. (2014). HIV, high school, and human rights: Putting faces on the failure to protect HIV + youth from bullying and discrimination at school. *University of La Verne Law Review, 35*(2), 267.

Grisso, T., & Appelbaum, P. S. (1998a). *MacArthur competence assessment tool for treatment (MacCAT–T)*. Sarasota, FL: Professional Resource Press.

Grisso, T., & Appelbaum, P. S. (1998b). *Assessing competence to consent to treatment*. New York: Oxford University Press.

Grisso, T., Appelbaum, P. S., & Hill-Fotouhi, C. (1997). The MacCAT–T: A clinical tool to assess patients' capacities to make treatment decisions. *Psychiatric Services, 48*, 1415–1419. doi:10.1176/ps.48.11.1415

Health Insurance Portability and Accountability Act of 1996 (HIPAA). (1996). P.L. no. 104–191, 110 Stat. 1938.

HIV Medicine Association. (2012). HIVMA urges repeal of HIV-specific criminal statutes. Available at http://www.hivma.org/uploadedFiles/HIVMA/FINAL%20HIVMA%20Policy% 20Statement%20on%20HIV%20Criminalization.pdf

Individuals with Disabilities Education Act (IDEA). (1990). P.L. no. 101–476, 104 Stat. 1142.

Individuals with Disabilities Education Act (IDEA). (2004). 20 U.S.C. Section 1400.

Kohlberg, L. (1984). *The psychology of moral development: The nature and validity of moral stages. Essays on moral development* (Vol. 2). New York: Harper & Row.

Larson, L. K. (2015). Employee health–AIDS discrimination. In M. Bender (Ed.), *Larson on employment discrimination* (Vol. 10, p. 170).

Marhefka, S. L., Turner, D., & Chenneville, T. (2017). HIV disclosure in pediatric populations: Who, what, when to tell, and then what?. In T. Chenneville (Ed.), A clinical guide to pediatric HIV: Bridging the gaps between research and practice. New York: Springer.

Marhefka, S. L., Valentin, C. R., Pinto, R. M., Demetriou, N., Wiznia, A., & Mellins, C. (2011). I feel like I'm carrying a weapon. Information and motivations related to sexual risk among girls with perinatally acquired HIV. *AIDS Care, 23*, 1321–1328. doi:10.1080/09540121.2010. 532536

Masty, J., & Fisher, C. (2008). A goodness-of-fit approach to informed consent for pediatric intervention research. *Ethics and Behavior, 18*(2–3), 139–160.

Moore, Q. L., Paul, M. E., McGuire, A. L., & Majumder, M. A. (2016). Legal barriers to adolescent participation in research about HIV and other sexually transmitted infections. *American Journal of Public Health, 106*(1), 40–44. doi:10.2105/AJPH.2015.302940

Murry, V. M., Berkel, C., Chen, Y. F., Brody, G. H., Gibbons, F. X., & Gerrard, M. (2011). Intervention induced changes on parenting practices, youth self-pride and sexual norms to reduce HIV-related behaviors among rural African American youths. *Journal of Youth and Adolescence, 40*(9), 1147–1163.

Mustanski, B., & Fisher, C. B. (2016). HIV rates are increasing in gay/bisexual teens: IRB barriers to research must be resolved to bend the curve. *American Journal of Preventive Medicine.* doi:10.1016/j.amepre.2016.02.026

Nagy, T. F. (2011). *Essential ethics for psychologists: A primer for understanding and mastering core issues.* Washington, DC: American Psychological Association. doi:10.1037/12345-000

National Commission for the Protection of Human Subjects of Biomedical and Behavioral Research. (1979). *The Belmont report: Ethical principles and guidelines for the protection of human subjects of research.* Washington, DC: National Institutes of Health.

National Conference of State Legislatures. (2016). State policies on sex education in schools. Retrieved from http://www.ncsl.org/research/health/state-policies-on-sex-education-in-schools. aspx

National Institutes of Health. (1949). Nuremberg code. Retrieved May 26, 2016, from https://history.nih.gov/research/downloads/nuremberg.pdf

Nichols, S. (2017). Developmental considerations for children and youth with HIV. In T. Chenneville (Ed.), *A clinical guide to pediatric HIV: Bridging the gaps between research and practice.* New York: Springer.

O'Byrne, P. (2012). Criminal law and public health practice: Are the Canadian HIV disclosure laws an effective HIV prevention strategy? *Sexuality Research and Social Policy, 7*(1), 70–79. doi:10.1007/s13178-011-0053-2

Paasche-Orlow, M. (2004). The ethics of cultural competence. *Academic Medicine, 79*(4), 347–350. doi:10.1097/00001888-200404000-00012

Public Welfare General Requirements for Informed Consent. (2003). 45 C.F.R. Section 46.116.

Rehabilitation Act of 1973. (1973). P. L. no. 93–112, 87 Stat. 355.

Sahay, S. (2013). Coming of age with HIV: A need for disclosure of HIV diagnosis among children/adolescents. *Journal of HIV/AIDS and Infectious Diseases, 1,* 1–7. doi:10.17303/jaid. 2013.103

Tarasoff v. Regents of the University of California. (1976, 1974). 17 Cal.3d 425, 551 P.2d 334.

World Medical Association. (2004). Declaration of Helsinki: Ethical principles for medical research involving human subjects. Retrieved May 27, 2016, from http://www.wma.net/en/30publications/10policies/b3/17c.pdf

Chapter 7
Catastrophic Consequences: The Link Between Rural Opioid Use and HIV/AIDS

Jennifer D. Lenardson and Mary Lindsey Smith

Introduction

Since the beginning of the HIV/AIDS epidemic, HIV transmission has been associated with drug abuse and addiction (National Institute on Drug Abuse, 2012). High-risk drug injection practices (e.g., sharing needles) and high-risk sexual behaviors (e.g., unprotected sex) are risk factors for HIV transmission and other blood borne diseases and these practices occur with the same or greater frequency in rural areas as they do in urban areas (Anderson, Wilson, Doll, Jones, & Barker, 1999; Lenardson, 2016a, b). Additionally, rural persons are more likely to live within closely tied social structures (Keyes, Cerda, Brady, Havens, & Galea, 2014), which have been associated with increased transmission rates (Draus & Carlson, 2009), and rural residents appear to have lower perceived risks of contracting HIV (Wright et al., 2014) and the negative consequences associated with heroin use (Lenardson, Gale, & Ziller, 2016). While HIV rates are typically lower in rural communities compared to urban areas, the growth in nonmedical opioid pain relievers and heroin among rural persons may lead to increased transmission of HIV in rural settings. In fact, 220 U.S. counties have been identified as potentially

J.D. Lenardson (✉)
Maine Rural Health Research Center, University of Southern Maine,
34 Bedford Street, 432B Wishcamper Center, Portland, ME 04104, USA
e-mail: Jennifer.lenardson@maine.edu

M.L. Smith
Maine Rural Health Research Center, University of Southern Maine,
34 Bedford Street, 410 Wishcamper Center, Portland, ME 04104, USA
e-mail: m.lindsey.smith@maine.edu

© Springer International Publishing AG 2017
F.M. Parks et al. (eds.), *HIV/AIDS in Rural Communities*,
DOI 10.1007/978-3-319-56239-1_7

vulnerable to an HIV or hepatitis C outbreak among persons who inject drugs and most of these counties are rural and over half (56%) are located in Kentucky, Tennessee, and West Virginia (Van Handel et al., 2016).

This chapter compares the prevalence of HIV and opioid use,[1] HIV and opioid treatment, and harm reduction in rural versus urban areas and presents information on state and local efforts to control HIV and opioid use in rural communities. In some cases, we describe hepatitis C and other types of substance use where the literature does not specifically address HIV or opioids.

Prevalence of Rural Opioid Abuse and HIV

Opioid use and HIV rates are lower among rural persons when compared to individuals residing in urban areas, however, some HIV risk factors and socio-demographic vulnerabilities are higher among rural persons. For example, research indicates that rural persons are more likely to engage in high-risk sexual behavior and are less likely to believe that there is any risk associated with trying heroin once or twice. Additionally, injection drug use practices which place individuals at high-risk for blood–borne disease transmission are similar between rural and urban persons who have used opioids in the past year.

Prevalence of Rural Opioid Use and User Characteristics

Multiple studies document higher nonmedical use of pain relievers among specific vulnerable rural populations, particularly among youth (Hartley, 2007; Havens, Young, & Havens, 2011), women who are pregnant (Shannon, Havens, & Hays, 2010) or experiencing partner violence (Cole & Logan, 2010), persons with co-occurring disorders (Kapoor & Thorn, 2014), and felony probationers (Havens, Oser, & Leukefeld, 2011; Havens et al., 2007). Studies show that nonmedical use of opioid pain relievers precedes heroin use, which is a cheaper and more accessible alternative to prescription opioids (Cicero, Ellis, Surratt, & Kurtz, 2014; Palamar, Shearston, Dawson, Mateu-Gelabert, & Ompad, 2016). Compared to heroin users 50 years ago, today's heroin users primarily live outside of urban areas (Cicero et al., 2014). In a national analysis examining the characteristics of opioid users, rural opioid users were more likely to have socioeconomic vulnerabilities that might put them at risk of adverse outcomes as a result of their drug use, including limited educational attainment, poor health status, being uninsured, and having low income (Lenardson et al., 2016).

---

[1]Consistent with current usage, we use the term "opioid" to refer to nonmedical opioid pain relievers and heroin.

Prevalence of HIV Among Rural Opioid Users

HIV prevalence data specific to rural persons who use opioids is limited and is approximated based on data available for injection drug use as a risk factor for HIV, state-specific studies, and rates of other blood–borne illnesses. Given that injection drug use is a risk factor for HIV (National Institute on Drug Abuse, 2012), the growth in opioids and injection use by persons living in rural communities will likely lead to an increase in HIV rates among this population. Nationally, persons who inject drugs represented a relatively small portion of new HIV infections—8% in 2010, 15% of those living with HIV in 2011 (National Center for HIV/AIDS, Viral Hepatitis, Sexual Transmitted Diseases and Tuberculosis Prevention, 2015b), and 20% of overall rural AIDS cases in 2009 (Health Resources and Services Administration, 2009). However, in 2014, the percent of diagnoses among males who obtained their HIV infection through injection drug use was slightly higher in nonmetropolitan areas (7%), than small (6%) and large (4%) metropolitan areas (National Center for HIV/AIDS, Viral Hepatitis, Sexual Transmitted Diseases, and Tuberculosis Prevention, 2014). Additionally, hepatitis B and C infections have grown in rural states and other rural settings in recent years, largely driven by prescription opioid abuse (Harris et al., 2016; Suryaprasad et al., 2014). The full impact of injection drug use on HIV prevalence is likely unknown given that surveillance and screening programs may underestimate HIV and hepatitis C prevalence as a result of access to care barriers, concerns with confidentiality, and stigma (Suryaprasad et al., 2014).

In drug-using communities, injection drug use is relatively widespread. Among methadone maintenance treatment enrollees located in 33 states, one-third of those who primarily abused prescription opioids reported that they had a lifetime history of injecting opioids, while 78% of those who primarily abused heroin had a lifetime history of injecting heroin (Rosenblum et al., 2007). However, national estimates from 2008 to 2014 found no statistical difference between rural and urban opioid users in reported prevalence of ever using a needle to inject drugs or ever using a needle to inject heroin (Fig. 7.1) (Lenardson, 2016a, b).

High-Risk Injection Drug Use Practices

Sterile syringes, needles, and other works are important in preventing persons who inject drugs from contracting HIV and hepatitis C (Division of AIDS Prevention, 2016; National Center for HIV/AIDS, Viral Hepatitis, Sexual Transmitted Diseases, and Tuberculosis Prevention, 2015a). However, high-risk injection drug practices are common among rural and urban persons who use opioids. Persons who inject drugs are unlikely to use sterile equipment; regardless of residence, a large proportion of all opioid users reused their own or someone else's needle and about three-quarters did not clean their needle with bleach before use (Fig. 7.2) (Lenardson, 2016a, b).

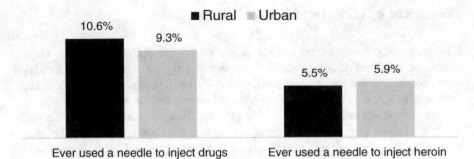

Fig. 7.1 Rural and urban opioid users inject drugs in similar proportions. *Data* National Survey of Drug Use and Health, 2008–2014. Residence differences not significant

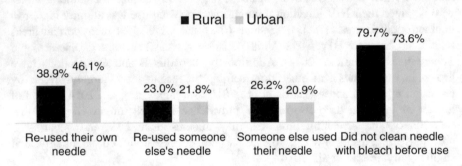

Fig. 7.2 Rural and urban opioid users engage in risky injection drug practices. *Data* National Survey of Drug Use and Health, 2008–2014. Residence differences not significant

Persons who inject opioid pain relievers in rural Appalachian Kentucky commonly reported cleaning their works with water only (Havens, Walker, & Leukefeld, 2007) or sharing their needles with others (Havens et al., 2011a). Additionally, those who reported sharing syringes in the past 6 months were more than twice as likely to have hepatitis C compared to those who did not share syringes (Havens et al., 2013). These high-risk injection drug practices along with other risky behaviors associated with substance use, place opioid users at increased risk for contracting HIV.

Risk of HIV Transmission from Sexual Behaviors

In addition to the dangers associated with high-risk injection drug practices, the use of injection drugs can increase sexual risk behaviors as a result of reduced inhibitions (National Center for HIV/AIDS, Viral Hepatitis, Sexual Transmitted Diseases and Tuberculosis Prevention, 2015a). In small-area studies, rural drug users reported sexual behavior magnifying their risk of HIV and other STDs. Nearly all stimulant[2] users across three rural North Carolina counties reported risk of HIV transmission and other STDs based on their sexual behavior, including sex while using drugs, sex trading, group sex, and not using condoms (Zule et al., 2007). The majority of current and former stimulant users in rural Arkansas, Kentucky, and Ohio used condoms inconsistently over a three-year period, while stimulant users who also used nonprescribed opioids had greater odds of engaging with multiple sexual partners (Borders et al., 2013). In three studies, examining sexual risk behaviors among rural probationers and incarcerated populations, participants reported high rates of unprotected sexual activity, and injection drug use (Leukefeld et al., 2003; Oser, Leukefeld, Cosentino-Boehm, & Havens, 2006; Staton-Tindall et al., 2015). These findings indicate that persons who use opioids engage in sexual behaviors that place them at increased risk for the transmission of HIV.

There are no recent national examinations of rural–urban differences in HIV transmission risk as a result of sexual behavior, however, national data through 1996 indicate that condom use was greater in urban areas (Anderson et al., 1999). Within rural communities in Kentucky and Florida, probationers and drug users reported high rates of unprotected sex and the exchange of sex for drugs or money (Brown & Van Hook, 2006; Crosby, Oser, Leukefeld, Havens, & Young, 2012; Oser et al., 2006). Given these limited data, condom use in rural areas may be lower among persons at risk for HIV as a result of drug use or other socio-demographic factors.

Social Networks as a Risk Factor for Virus Transmission

In a literature review, Keyes et al. noted that rural social networks are more closely tied than urban social networks (Keyes et al., 2014). The combination of small social circles, limited economic opportunities, lack of substance use disorder treatment, and abundant drug supplies may magnify the use of drugs and risk of HIV in rural areas (Draus & Carlson, 2009). Among persons who used drugs in rural Appalachian Kentucky, nearly two-thirds of the sample were linked by a sexual relationship to another person within the sample (Crosby et al., 2012). Additionally, among high-risk rural drug users in Appalachia, a member of the main group of rural drug users with HIV was predicted to spread the infection to 18% of the rest of the sample (Young, Jonas, Mullins, Halgin, & Havens, 2013). Evidence of how these close social networks can contribute to the transmission of HIV occurred in Scott County, Indiana, a small community of just 4,200 people, where 135 were diagnosed with HIV in 2015. The majority (80%) of those newly infected reported injection of the prescription opioid oxymorphone and 84% were co-infected with the hepatitis C virus. Among this network of newly identified HIV

---

[2]Stimulants are a class of drugs that increase attention, alertness, and energy and elevate heart rate and blood pressure. Prescription stimulants are often used to treat attention deficit hyperactivity disorder; in the study cited here (Zule et al., 2007), stimulants refers to powder cocaine, crack, and methamphetamine.

patients, 230 social contacts were tested, identifying an additional 109 HIV-positive people (Morbidity and Mortality Weekly Report, 2015). Given the closely tied social networks in rural communities coupled with the interconnectedness of sexual relationships between persons who use drugs in rural areas, it is likely that this population is at increased risk of exposure and transmission of HIV. The risk of transmission is further exacerbated by rural residents' low perception of risk of contracting HIV.

Lower Perceived Risk Among Rural Persons

In general, rural residents appear to have a low perception of HIV and heroin risk, especially in comparison to urban residents. In a national study, rural heroin users were less likely than urban users to say there was a great risk associated with trying heroin only once or twice (41% vs. 54.4%); in particular, rural males were less likely to perceive a great risk (Lenardson et al., 2016). Research also indicates that specific subpopulations of rural residents have a low perception of HIV risk. For example, among low-income African American drug-using women in Missouri, rural women were twice as likely as urban women to say they did not receive HIV counseling during their last pregnancy, their sex partner had not been tested for HIV, and they did not use HIV prevention methods or condoms because they did not worry about infection (Crosby et al., 2012). Moreover, among rural African American cocaine users in Arkansas, over half believed they were not at risk of acquiring HIV despite cocaine use, multiple sex partners, and inconsistent condom use (Wright et al., 2014). African American cocaine users in the Arkansas Delta also expressed the erroneous belief that they had received an HIV test during routine appointments even though they had not been informed about a test and they assumed the results were negative because they had never received results (Wright, Stewart, Curran, & Booth, 2013). Rural opioid users have a low perception of risk from heroin and rural African American women who use drugs have a low perception of HIV risk.

Though opioid use and HIV rates are lower among rural residents compared to urban, several HIV risk factors and socio-demographic vulnerabilities are higher among rural persons. For example, hepatitis B and C infections have grown in rural states and other rural settings in recent years, largely driven by prescription opioid abuse, while needle sharing and unsanitary needle practices do not differ between rural and urban persons who use opioids. Based on the results of small area studies that indicate high-risk sexual behavior among rural drug users, we suspect that unprotected sex may be higher in rural areas than urban. Close social networks in rural communities and a low perception of HIV and heroin risk may facilitate increased exposure and transmission of HIV.

HIV and Opioid Treatment

Treatment for substance use disorders can be an important component of HIV prevention. People who receive treatment for substance use disorders often receive HIV risk reduction messages, an effective tool in stopping or reducing drug use and related risk behaviors such as unsafe sex and injection practices (National Institute on Drug Abuse, 2012). The availability of general treatment for substance use disorders and treatment specifically targeting opioid use disorders is limited in rural areas. Additionally, where treatment services are available, specialty options such as medication-assisted therapy may be unavailable. Rural–urban quality of care comparisons are not available for HIV patients who also have a comorbid diagnosis of substance use disorder, therefore, we present a review of the current data on the availability of opioid and HIV treatment options as well as a summary of the barriers associated with accessing care for opioid dependence and HIV in rural areas.

Availability of Opioid Treatment

The availability of opioid use treatment programs in rural communities is limited and access to treatment for individuals with HIV/AIDS is rare in rural areas. As of 2011,[3] only 7% of all opioid treatment programs (OTPs)—programs that use methadone and other medications to treat heroin and other opioid use disorders—were located in rural areas. Among substance use treatment facilities offering treatment programs specifically for persons with HIV/AIDS, 10% were located in rural areas in 2011 (Lenardson, 2016a, b). Out of the 85 treatment facilities across the country offering both OTPs and programs for persons with HIV/AIDS, only 11 were located in rural areas (Lenardson, 2016a, b). The number of OTPs in urban counties providing buprenorphine was 11.4 for every one program in a rural county in 2011, while the number of substance abuse facilities providing buprenorphine was 9.5 in urban counties compared to every one in a rural county (Stein et al., 2015). Nearly all (90%) office-based physicians who hold a waiver from the Drug Enforcement Administration to prescribe buprenorphine–naloxone for opioid use disorder practice in urban counties (Rosenblatt et al., 2015). The limited supply of OTPs in rural areas could be related to the need for an adequate supply of patients to fund these type of comprehensive programs as well as perceived lack of privacy for specialty substance abuse treatment in rural areas (Fortney et al., 2004). The urban location of OTPs may deter treatment for rural patients since opioid treatments are typically dispensed on a daily basis, requiring prohibitive travel (Mann & Edwards, 2004). Additionally, rural areas may have difficulty recruiting specialty providers to staff these programs.

---

[3]Though more recent data are available from the National Survey of Substance Abuse Treatment Services, these data do not include an indicator of rural–urban facility location and we were required to use the last known available dataset with this variable.

In a national sample of substance use treatment facilities, rural facilities were more likely to provide specialized adolescent treatment than urban centers and more likely to have nursing staff, however, they were less likely to offer buprenorphine, had fewer wraparound services, and offered less diverse specialized treatment options (Edmond, Aletraris, & Roman, 2015). In some rural populations, associated use of benzodiazepines and prescription opioids is common, yet few methadone clinics have the capacity to handle detoxification and treatment for these two drugs in combination (Havens et al., 2007). Availability of OTPs in rural areas is limited and the specialized combination of OTP and HIV care are likely to be unusual in rural areas, requiring travel to urban areas for services or use of separate HIV and substance use disorder programs. Telehealth applications may help rural persons bridge the gap between residence and location of specialty treatment programs. Small-scale demonstrations of telehealth applications have successfully implemented adjunct substance use disorder treatment services such as disease self-management and assessment among veterans (Santa Ana, Stallings, Rounsaville, & Martino, 2013) and medication adherence among persons with HIV/AIDS (Tucker, Simpson, Huang, Roth, & Stewart, 2013). Although technological applications present promising options for the future of substance use disorder treatment and management, at present access and availability to treatment programs remain the principle barriers to treatment for individuals living in rural areas.

Quality of HIV Care for Rural Persons Who Inject Drugs

Several studies have shown negative outcomes associated with rural location of HIV patients or providers, such as delayed entry into treatment, reduced odds of receiving highly active antiretroviral therapy (HAART), and an increased mortality rate in national (Cohn et al., 2001; Ohl et al., 2010) and state-specific studies (Day, Conroy, Lowe, Page, & Dolan, 2006; Lahey et al., 2007; Sheehan et al., 2015). In a consortium of 21 sites that provide HIV care, persons living with HIV/AIDS in rural areas who received care in urban areas received appropriate levels of opportunistic infection prophylaxis and HAART use. Rural patients had lower inpatient and outpatient use than urban patients though they were just as likely to obtain virologic suppression. Persons who injected drugs were 19% less likely to receive HAART than those who did not inject drugs (Wilson et al., 2011). Site of care may be a determining factor in quality of HIV care. When rural patients travel to urban sites to receive care or when urban providers travel to rural sites to deliver care, high-quality HIV care has been attained (Wilson et al., 2011).

Studies have shown that medication-assisted therapy successfully decreased risk factors among persons who inject drugs and improved quality of life for HIV patients, however, comparisons between rural–urban patients or clinics were not examined (Korthuis et al., 2011; Sorensen & Copeland, 2000). Additionally, treatment of opioid dependence with methadone or buprenorphine is associated with reduced drug use and reduced high-risk sex and injection drug practices (Gowing, Hickman, & Degenhardt, 2013). Although these therapies represent a potential solution to some of the barriers to accessing quality care for individuals with opioid use disorders and HIV, further research is needed to explore how medication-assisted therapy in rural areas can reduce treatment barriers and increase access and quality of care.

Barriers to Treatment

Barriers to substance use disorder and HIV treatment specific to rural persons include transportation and distance, discrimination, stigma, confidentiality concerns exacerbated by small town settings, and limited public and private health insurance coverage for substance use disorders.

Travel and Distance Barriers

In general, travel and distance are commonly identified barriers to healthcare access for rural residents (Ziller, Lenardson, & Coburn, 2012). Given the specialty nature of both substance use disorder and HIV services, travel and distance are also rural barriers for these forms of care. Patients who live in low or moderately populated counties travel longer distances to an OTP than patients in more densely populated counties (Rosenblum et al., 2011). Among HIV patients living in New Hampshire, rural patients had significantly longer travel time to HIV care than urban patients (56 vs. 34 minutes) (Lahey et al., 2007). In a survey of rural county health departments in 10 southern states, the average distance to reach HIV treatment sites was over 50 miles (Sutton, Anthony, Vila, McLellan-Lemal, & Weidle, 2010). In the face of a hypothetical preventive HIV vaccine, rural men who used drugs in Appalachian Kentucky identified time to visit a clinic as a barrier to vaccine acceptability (Young, DiClemente, Halgin, Sterk, & Havens, 2014). Distance and transportation to substance use disorder and HIV services continues to be a significant barrier for individuals living in rural communities. National efforts to integrate medication-assisted treatment into a variety of medical settings, including primary care clinics, may increase rural residents' access to these services.

Discrimination, Stigma, and Confidentiality Barriers

Several small area, qualitative studies have found that rural persons who use injection drugs or rural persons with HIV experience discrimination or stigma in accessing health care. In rural Oregon, HIV-positive patients reported healthcare providers who were afraid to touch them, who discouraged or refused treatment, and who posed

intrusive or rude questions (Zukoski & Thorburn, 2009). These experiences negatively impacted the HIV-positive patients who reacted with anger, discouragement,
shame, isolation, and decisions not to disclose their status in the future (Zukoski &
Thorburn, 2009). In addition, perceived stigma has been found to be negatively
associated with quality of life among HIV-positive individuals living in rural southeastern states (Vyavaharkar, Moneyham, Murdaugh, & Tavakoli, 2012).

Research indicates that stigma and discrimination among rural injection drug users
can contribute to risky drug use practices and place drug users at increased risk for
exposure and transmission of HIV. For example, Project Lazarus, a community-based
opioid intervention in rural North Carolina, found that trying to identify legitimate and
illicit users only exacerbated stigma and stopped those at greatest risk from receiving
prevention messages and an overdose antidote (Albert et al., 2011).

In an examination of HIV-related depression, stigma, and anxiety in North
Carolina, rural participants reported greater disclosure concerns than urban participants (Costelloe et al., 2015). Rural persons were concerned for their confidentiality
when receiving HIV and behavioral health care at facilities where friends and relatives
worked (Duran et al., 2005; Wright et al., 2013). When compared to individuals living
in urban areas, rural persons were more likely to identify negative reactions from
family and employers as a primary reason why they felt uncomfortable receiving
substance use disorder treatment (Davis, 2009). Stigma, discrimination, and confidentiality concerns can serve as barriers to HIV and substance use disorder treatment
for rural persons who live in small communities with less anonymity.

Insurance Barriers

Compared to urban persons who used opioids in the past year, rural persons were
more likely to be uninsured or publicly insured and less likely to have private
insurance (Fig. 7.3) (Lenardson, 2016a, b). Furthermore, even when persons who
use opioids had access to health insurance coverage, they were likely to encounter

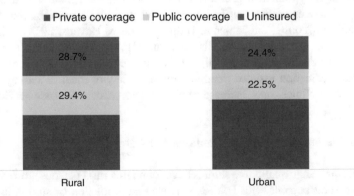

Fig. 7.3 Rural opioid users are more likely to be publicly insured or uninsured. *Data* National
Survey of Drug Use and Health, 2008–2014. Residence differences not significant *p* < 0.001

treatment limits. For instance, in 2013, only 13 state Medicaid programs covered all medications approved for opioid dependence on their approved drug lists. Nearly, all state Medicaid programs required prior approval for buprenorphine–naloxone, while 11 programs placed 1–3-year lifetime treatment limits on these medications (Mark, Lubran, McCance-Katz, Chalk, & Richardson, 2015). Private health insurers also limit substance use disorder treatment coverage. After patients with private insurance were hospitalized for opioid misuse, only 11% received the recommended combination of medication and therapeutic services, while 40% did not receive any follow-up services within a month after their hospitalization (Ali & Mutter, 2013). Neither public nor private insurance provides the ongoing treatment and chronic disease management necessary for long-term recovery.

Harm Reduction

Harm reduction in substance use disorder treatment is a nonabstinence-based intervention that seeks to eliminate the negative consequences of substance use disorders for those willing to be in treatment, even if they are not yet ready to abstain from drug use. While previous programs and policies have focused on abstinence, many of the consequences of drug use—including HIV and hepatitis C—can be reduced or eliminated without complete abstinence through evidence-based harm reduction activities, such as methadone maintenance treatment or syringe exchange programs (MacMaster, 2004; van den Berg, Smit, van Brussel, Coutinho, & Prins, 2007). However, in international, national, and state-specific studies, when compared to urban areas, rural areas were less likely to receive harm reduction services.

Syringe Exchange Programs

In December 2015, President Obama's bipartisan budget agreement lifted the federal ban on federal funds to support syringe exchange programs (SEPs) (Office of the Press Secretary, 2016). SEPs are community-based programs that provide access and disposal of sterile needles and syringes and are typically part of a larger, comprehensive approach to HIV prevention that includes prevention materials (e.g., sterile water, condoms, alcohol swabs), education on safer injection practices and wound care, overdose prevention, referral to substance use and HIV/hepatitis C treatment, and counseling and testing for HIV/hepatitis C (Division of AIDS Prevention, 2016). Most SEPs also encourage secondary exchange, where persons attending the program exchange needles for peers who do not attend (Des Jarlais et al., 2015). In a 2013 national survey of 295 SEPs, the majority of programs (78%) were located in a suburban or urban location, only 20% were located in rural areas, with the West and Midwest representing the greatest proportion of rural programs. Rural SEPs exchanged fewer syringes than suburban and urban programs (2.7 million for rural

SEPS compared to 35.9 million for suburban and urban) and had more modest budgets. However, based on this analysis, it is unclear if there were rural residents who need SEP services but were going without compared to urban residents.

Limited research suggests that rural persons who inject drugs have inadequate access to SEPs. In a convenience sample of people who inject drugs living in rural and urban areas of Connecticut, rural persons were not accessing SEPs, which was attributed to limited hours of operation, limited geographic access, and lack of program awareness in rural areas (Grau, Zhan, & Heimer, 2016). Rural drug users in Canada and Australia were less likely than urban users to use a SEP as their usual source of injection equipment and were more likely to use pharmacies and other users for their equipment compared to urban users (Day et al., 2006; Parker, Jackson, Dykeman, Gahagan, & Karabanow, 2012). When they were able to attend a SEP, rural Canadian users obtained their own supply of needles and a supply for nonattending peers as well as food, a place to launder clothing, and referrals for other services (Parker et al., 2012). These international SEPs have innovative features including delivery by urban programs to rural participants in Canada and vending machine delivery of needles in Australia. In sum, rural persons who use injection drugs may face several barriers to using SEPs, including their limited presence in rural communities and few treatment options for participants who are ready for recovery. Implications for improving access include making these services available through existing programs (e.g., public health departments or local hospitals) or through mobile vans or home delivery.

Safe Injection Facilities and Heroin Maintenance

In recent years, Canada has introduced both a safe injection facility and a heroin maintenance program in Vancouver, though it seems unlikely that these programs will become available in the U.S. Safe injection facilities are nurse-supervised drug injection sites where clients are provided with sterile equipment and an opportunity to connect with primary healthcare and treatment services. Safe injection facilities have been associated with reductions in needle sharing. For example, in Vancouver, a safe injection facility was used to reduce syringe sharing among injection drug users which helped to stem an unprecedented outbreak of HIV in Vancouver (Kerr, Tyndall, Li, Montaner, & Wood, 2005; O'Shaughnessy, Hogg, Strathdee, & Montaner, 2012). A first in the U.S., Ithaca, New York has proposed a similar safe injection facility as a way to connect heroin users to treatment and to protect against overdose fatalities (Foderaro, 2016). A prescription heroin maintenance program in Vancouver reduced use and costs associated with jail, emergency rooms, and other social services. The program targets a select group of patients who have attempted other heroin maintenance programs and replacement therapy programs (Levin, 2016). Small, rural U.S. communities with less bureaucracy and closely tied social networks may have an advantage in attempting to operationalize these novel programs as alternatives to medical treatment and criminal prosecution.

State and Local Treatment Efforts with Rural Relevance

Pioneering state and local treatment models have relevance for rural communities and address shortcomings of existing services, such as delivering treatment via telehealth application or through a nonsubstance or HIV associated provider to build on existing service providers and address confidentiality concerns. State and local efforts to treat and limit the spread of infectious disease among persons who use drugs and other high-risk persons include prevention and harm reduction, use of innovative counseling approaches, an integrated treatment model for HIV and substance use disorders model, a comprehensive public health approach to an HIV outbreak, and a blended model of rural–urban HIV treatment. After a hepatitis B outbreak in the late 2000s, Tennessee worked with county jails to increase hepatitis B vaccination coverage among incarcerated persons, while West Virginia began a training program collaboration with addiction centers and harm reduction programs to prevent hepatitis B (Harris et al., 2016). Resource constraints in rural communities suggest the need for collaboration across concerned parties.

In an assessment of church-based religious support on sexual risk behaviors in rural, impoverished counties in the Arkansas and Mississippi Delta region, positive religious coping (collaborative problem-solving, positive reappraisals, and benevolent religious involvement) was associated with fewer sexual encounters and partners for African Americans who used cocaine (Montgomery et al., 2014). Programs targeting African Americans in the South may be especially important given that this population group is disproportionately impacted by HIV. In a national study of veterans with HIV, rural veterans had substituted primary care for infectious disease treatment mainly as a result of distance. Improved models of telehealth were suggested to overcome these geographic barriers to specialty treatment programs (Ohl, Richardson, Kaboli, Perencevich, & Vaughan-Sarrazin, 2014). Telehealth applications, such as interactive voice response systems, have been useful in assessing medication adherence in rural persons living with HIV/AIDS in Alabama. This system was also used to track risk behaviors, such as alcohol and drug use, sexual activity, and sexual risk behaviors (Tucker et al., 2013).

Health Services Center, Inc. (HSC) of Anniston, Alabama provides care to people with HIV/AIDS who use drugs or have a history of drug use. To overcome distance and transportation barriers, HSC provides primary care, mental health and substance use disorder treatment, case management, and free medication onsite as well through a mobile clinic and home visiting service across 14 rural counties with five satellite offices. HSC maintains a harm reduction focus for its substance use disorder treatment services and offers three levels of HIV treatment adherence intervention based on clients' needs. Outreach is provided to multiple community groups including a juvenile detention center, a domestic violence center, churches, self-help and civic programs, an outpatient substance abuse treatment program, and a palliative care program (Wood, 2008).

To reduce communicable disease and serve as a pathway to drug treatment, the Cabell-Huntington Harm Reduction and Needle Exchange Program in Appalachian

West Virginia provides needles, syringes and sterile water, cotton filters, cookers, and alcohol swabs and condoms at no charge to 150 heroin users each week since opening in September 2015. The weekly clinic also offers free screening for HIV, hepatitis, and STDs, as well as pregnancy tests, contraceptive services, and first aid for wounds and instruction on and distribution of naloxone. The program features a recovery coach, a peer in recovery who helps someone new to treatment understand the process. Attendees are also encouraged to use the health department's primary care and chronic disease management services. Unfortunately, a lack of medication-assisted treatment in the area limits options when patients are ready to seek treatment (Vestal, 2016).

Another program aimed at limiting the spread of blood–borne diseases was established in Indiana after an outbreak of HIV in Scott County among its community of injection opioid users. The Indiana State Department of Health's comprehensive response included a public education campaign, a community outreach center, short-term authorization of syringe exchange and support for comprehensive medical care for HIV and hepatitis C as well as substance use disorder treatment and counseling (Morbidity and Mortality Weekly Report, 2015). Since July of 2015, the state's comprehensive response appears to be slowing the spread of further transmissions, with only 14 new cases of HIV and viral suppression of 50% of existing cases (Rudavsky, 2016).

Some states have established programs to improve access to HIV treatment services and experienced specialty providers in rural areas. For example, Vermont has implemented a rural HIV service delivery model that provides care at rural regional hospitals staffed by a HIV-trained nurse practitioner and social worker, while a University of Vermont infectious disease physician visits each clinic monthly. In between physician visits, care is provided by a nurse practitioner and reviewed by telephone with the physician. Rural and urban patients were found to have no differences in viral suppression, rise in median CD4 counts over time, or survival (Grace et al., 2010).

Conclusion

Several factors conspire to make it difficult to examine opioid use and HIV status across the rural continuum. Despite prominence in news coverage and negative outcomes, the prevalence of opioid use and HIV status in the population is low, making it difficult to identify reportable differences in national data. Additionally, opioid use and HIV status are characteristics that require confidentiality among reporting systems. Rural–urban data on substance use and treatment facilities is often not released in public-use files because it could potentially identify its subjects. Obtaining a rural–urban indicator within the dataset may be available through a rigorous application procedure; however, this process does not lend itself to regular examination of trends among persons with both opioid use and HIV.

Several studies discussed here examine a specific rural community. Going forward, it will be important to supplement these studies with comparisons of rural and urban communities within the same state or featuring similar demographic features and nationwide to determine if the characteristics of rural persons who use opioids and are HIV-positive are different from urban persons and to examine rural and urban variations in access to treatment. Rural–urban quality of care comparisons are needed for HIV patients who also have a comorbid substance use disorder diagnosis.

References

Albert, S., Brason, F. W., Sanford, C. K., Dasgupta, N., Graham, J., & Lovette, B. (2011). Project Lazarus: Community-based overdose prevention in rural North Carolina. *Pain Medicine, 12*(suppl 2), S77–S85. doi:10.1111/j.1526-4637.2011.01128.x

Ali, M. M., & Mutter, R. (2013). Patients who are privately insured receive limited follow-up services after opioid-related hospitalizations. *The CBHSQ Report*. Rockville (MD).

Anderson, J. E., Wilson, R., Doll, L., Jones, T. S., & Barker, P. (1999). Condom use and HIV risk behaviors among U.S. adults: Data from a national survey. *Family Planning Perspectives, 31*(1), 24–28.

Borders, T. F., Stewart, K. E., Wright, P. B., Leukefeld, C., Falck, R. S., Carlson, R. G., & Booth, B. M. (2013). Risky sex in rural America: Longitudinal changes in a community-based cohort of methamphetamine and cocaine users. *American Journal on Addictions, 22*(6), 535–542. doi:10.1111/j.1521-0391.2013.12028.x

Brown, E. J., & Van Hook, M. (2006). Risk behavior, perceptions of HIV risk, and risk-reduction behavior among a small group of rural African American women who use drugs. *Journal of the Association of Nurses in AIDS Care, 17*(5), 42–50. doi:10.1016/j.jana.2006.07.004

Cicero, T. J., Ellis, M. S., Surratt, H. L., & Kurtz, S. P. (2014). The changing face of heroin use in the United States: A retrospective analysis of the past 50 years. *JAMA Psychiatry, 71*(7), 821–826. doi:10.1001/jamapsychiatry.2014.366

Cohn, S. E., Berk, M. L., Berry, S. H., Duan, N., Frankel, M. R., Klein, J. D., …, Bozzette, S. A. (2001). The care of HIV-infected adults in rural areas of the United States. *JAIDS Journal of Acquired Immune Deficiency Syndromes, 28*(4), 385–392.

Cole, J., & Logan, T. K. (2010). Nonmedical use of sedative-hypnotics and opiates among rural and urban women with protective orders. *Journal of Addictive Diseases, 29*(3), 395–409. doi:10.1080/10550887.2010.489453

Costelloe, S., Kemppainen, J., Brion, J., MacKain, S., Reid, P., Frampton, A., Rigsbee, E. (2015). Impact of anxiety and depressive symptoms on perceptions of stigma in persons living with HIV disease in rural versus urban North Carolina. *AIDS Care, 27*(12), 1425–1428. doi:10.1080/09540121.2015.1114993

Crosby, R. A., Oser, C. B., Leukefeld, C. G., Havens, J. R., & Young, A. (2012). Prevalence of HIV and risky sexual behaviors among rural drug users: Does age matter? *Annals of Epidemiology, 22*(11), 778–782. doi:10.1016/j.annepidem.2012.07.006

Davis, W. M. (2009). *Barriers to substance abuse treatment utilization in rural versus urban Pennsylvania (unpublished doctoral dissertation)*. Indiana, PA: Indiana University of Pennsylvania.

Day, C., Conroy, E., Lowe, J., Page, J., & Dolan, K. (2006). Patterns of drug use and associated harms among rural injecting drug users: Comparisons with metropolitan injecting drug users. *Australian Journal of Rural Health, 14*(3), 120–125. doi:10.1111/j.1440-1584.2006.00775.x

Des Jarlais, D. C., Nugent, A., Solberg, A., Feelemyer, J., Mermin, J., & Holtzman, D. (2015). Syringe service programs for persons who inject drugs in urban, suburban, and rural areas— United States, 2013. *MMWR: Morbidity and Mortality Weekly Report, 64*(48), 1337–1341. doi:10.15585/mmwr.mm6448a3

Division of AIDS Prevention. (2016). Syringe service programs. Retrieved from http://www.cdc.gov/hiv/risk/ssps.html

Draus, P., & Carlson, R. G. (2009). Down on main street: Drugs and the small-town vortex. *Health Place, 15*(1), 247–254. doi:10.1016/j.healthplace.2008.05.004

Duran, B., Oetzel, J., Lucero, J., Jiang, Y., Novins, D. K., Manson, S., Beals, J. (2005). Obstacles for rural American Indians seeking alcohol, drug, or mental health treatment. *Journal of Consulting and Clinical Psychology, 73*(5), 819–829. doi:10.1037/0022-006X.73.5.819

Edmond, M. B., Aletraris, L., & Roman, P. M. (2015). Rural substance use treatment centers in the United States: An assessment of treatment quality by location. *The American Journal of Drug and Alcohol Abuse, 41*(5), 449–457. doi:10.3109/00952990.2015.1059842

Foderaro, L. (2016, March 22). Fighting heroin, ithaca looks to injection centers. *The New York Times.*

Fortney, J., Mukherjee, S., Curran, G., Fortney, S., Han, X., & Booth, B. M. (2004). Factors associated with perceived stigma for alcohol use and treatment among at-risk drinkers. *Journal of Behavioral Health Services and Research, 31*(4), 418–429.

Gowing, L. R., Hickman, M., & Degenhardt, L. (2013). Mitigating the risk of HIV infection with opioid substitution treatment. *Bulletin of the World Health Organization, 91*(2), 81–156.

Grace, C., Kutzko, D., Alston, W. K., Ramundo, M., Polish, L., & Osler, T. (2010). The Vermont model for rural HIV care delivery: Eleven years of outcome data comparing urban and rural clinics. *Journal of Rural Health, 26*(2), 113–119. doi:10.1111/j.1748-0361.2010.00272.x

Grau, L. E., Zhan, W., & Heimer, R. (2016). Prevention knowledge, risk behaviours and seroprevalence among nonurban injectors of southwest Connecticut. *Drug and Alcohol Review.* doi:10.1111/dar.12396

Harris, A. M., Iqbal, K., Schillie, S., Britton, J., Kainer, M. A., Tressler, S., Vellozzi, C. (2016). Increases in acute hepatitis B virus infections—Kentucky, Tennessee, and West Virginia, 2006–2013. *MMWR: Morbidity and Mortality Weekly Report, 65*(3), 47–50. doi:10.15585/mmwr.mm6503a2

Hartley, D. (2007). *Substance abuse among rural youth: A little meth and a lot of booze* (Research and Policy Brief No. 35A). Retrieved from Portland, ME: http://muskie.usm.maine.edu/Publications/rural/pb35a.pdf

Havens, J. R., Lofwall, M. R., Frost, S. D., Oser, C. B., Leukefeld, C. G., & Crosby, R. A. (2013). Individual and network factors associated with prevalent hepatitis C infection among rural Appalachian injection drug users. *American Journal of Public Health, 103*(1), e44–e52. doi:10.2105/AJPH.2012.300874

Havens, J. R., Oser, C. B., & Leukefeld, C. G. (2011a). Injection risk behaviors among rural drug users: Implications for HIV prevention. *AIDS Care, 23*(5), 638–645. doi:10.1080/09540121.2010.516346

Havens, J. R., Oser, C. B., Leukefeld, C. G., Webster, J. M., Martin, S. S., O'Connell, D. J., … Inciardi, J. A. (2007). Differences in prevalence of prescription opiate misuse among rural and urban probationers. *American Journal of Drug and Alcohol Abuse, 33*(2), 309–317. doi:10.1080/00952990601175078

Havens, J. R., Walker, R., & Leukefeld, C. G. (2007b). Prevalence of opioid analgesic injection among rural nonmedical opioid analgesic users. *Drug and Alcohol Dependence, 87*(1), 98–102. doi:10.1016/j.drugalcdep.2006.07.008

Havens, J. R., Young, A. M., & Havens, C. E. (2011b). Nonmedical prescription drug use in a nationally representative sample of adolescents: Evidence of greater use among rural adolescents. *Archives of Pediatrics and Adolescent Medicine, 165*(3), 250–255. doi:10.1001/archpediatrics.2010.217

Health Resources and Services Administration. (2009). *HIV/AIDS in rural America*. Washington, DC: U.S. Department of Health and Human Services.

Kapoor, S., & Thorn, B. E. (2014). Healthcare use and prescription of opioids in rural residents with pain. *Rural and Remote Health, 14*(2879) (online).

Kerr, T., Tyndall, M., Li, K., Montaner, J., & Wood, E. (2005). Safer injection facility use and syringe sharing in injection drug users. *Lancet, 366*(9482), 316–318. doi:10.1016/S0140-6736(05)66475-6

Keyes, K. M., Cerda, M., Brady, J. E., Havens, J. R., & Galea, S. (2014). Understanding the rural-urban differences in nonmedical prescription opioid use and abuse in the United States. *American Journal of Public Health, 104*(2), e52–e59. doi:10.2105/AJPH.2013.301709

Korthuis, P. T., Tozzi, M. J., Nandi, V., Fiellin, D. A., Weiss, L., Egan, J. E., ... Collaborative, B. (2011). Improved quality of life for opioid-dependent patients receiving buprenorphine treatment in HIV clinics. *Journal of Acquired Immune Deficiency Syndromes, 56*(Suppl 1), S39–S45. doi:10.1097/QAI.0b013e318209754c

Lahey, T., Lin, M., Marsh, B., Curtin, J., Wood, K., Eccles, B., & von Reyn, C. F. (2007). Increased mortality in rural patients with HIV in New England. *AIDS Research and Human Retroviruses, 23*(5), 693–698. doi:10.1089/aid.2006.0206

Lenardson, J. D. (2016a). *Unpublished tabulations of the 2008–14 national survey of drug use and health*. Portland, ME: Maine Rural Health Research Center.

Lenardson, J. D. (2016b). *Unpublished tabulations of the national survey of substance abuse treatment services, 2011 and 2014*. Portland, ME: Maine Rural Health Research Center.

Lenardson, J. D., Gale, J. A., & Ziller, E. C. (2016). *Rural opioid abuse: Prevalence and user characteristics*. Portland, ME: Maine Rural Health Research Center.

Leukefeld, C., Roberto, H., Hiller, M., Webster, M., Logan, T. K., & Staton-Tindall, M. (2003). HIV prevention among high-risk and hard-to-reach rural residents. *Journal of Psychoactive Drugs, 35*(4), 427–434. doi:10.1080/02791072.2003.10400489

Levin, D. (2016, April 21). Vancouver Prescriptions for Addicts Gain Attention as Heroin and Opioid Use Rises. *The New York Times*.

MacMaster, S. A. (2004). Harm reduction: A new perspective on substance abuse services. *Social Work, 49*(3), 356–363 358. doi:sw/49.3.353

Mann, B. (Writer) & B. H. Edwards (Director). (2004). Profile: Methadone treatments for heroin addicts, *NPR Morning Edition* (Radio transcript)

Mark, T. L., Lubran, R., McCance-Katz, E. F., Chalk, M., & Richardson, J. (2015). Medicaid coverage of medications to treat alcohol and opioid dependence. *Journal of Substance Abuse Treatment, 55*, 1–5. doi:10.1016/j.jsat.2015.04.009

Montgomery, B. E., Stewart, K. E., Yeary, K. H., Cornell, C. E., Pulley, L., Corwyn, R., & Ounpraseuth, S. T. (2014). Religiosity and sexual risk behaviors among African American cocaine users in the rural South. *Journal of Rural Health, 30*(3), 284–291. doi:10.1111/jrh.12059

Morbidity and Mortality Weekly Report. (2015). *Community outbreak of HIV infection linked to injection drug use of oxymorphone—Indiana, 2015*. Atlanta, GA: Centers for Disease Control and Prevention.

National Center for HIV/AIDS, Viral Hepatitis, Sexual Transmitted Diseases and Tuberculosis Prevention. (2014). *Estimated numbers and percentage of diagnosis of HIV infection among adults and adolescents, Male by MSA, 2014-US*. Atlanta, GA: Centers for Disease Control and Prevention.

National Center for HIV/AIDS, Viral Hepatitis, Sexual Transmitted Diseases and Tuberculosis Prevention. (2015a). HIV and injection drug use in the United States. Retrieved from http://www.cdc.gov/hiv/risk/idu.html

National Center for HIV/AIDS, Viral Hepatitis, Sexual Transmitted Diseases and Tuberculosis Prevention. (2015b). HIV in the United States: At a glance. Retrieved from http://www.cdc.gov/hiv/statistics/overview/ataglance.html

National Institute on Drug Abuse. (2012). DRUGFACTS: HIV/AIDS and drug abuse: Intertwined epidemics. Retrieved from https://www.drugabuse.gov/publications/drugfacts/hivaids-drug-abuse-intertwined-epidemics

O'Shaughnessy, M. V., Hogg, R. S., Strathdee, S. A., & Montaner, J. S. (2012). Deadly public policy: What the future could hold for the HIV epidemic among injection drug users in Vancouver. Current HIV/AIDS Reports, 9(4), 394–400. doi:10.1007/s11904-012-0130-z

Office of the Press Secretary. (2016). Fact sheet: President Obama proposes $1.1 billion in new funding to address the prescription opioid abuse and heroin use epidemic (Press release).

Ohl, M., Tate, J., Duggal, M., Skanderson, M., Scotch, M., Kaboli, P., ... Justice, A. (2010). Rural residence is associated with delayed care entry and increased mortality among veterans with human immunodeficiency virus infection. Medical Care, 48(12), 1064–1070. doi:10.1097/MLR.0b013e3181ef60c2

Ohl, M. E., Richardson, K., Kaboli, P. J., Perencevich, E. N., & Vaughan-Sarrazin, M. (2014). Geographic access and use of infectious diseases specialty and general primary care services by veterans with HIV Infection: Implications for telehealth and shared care programs. The Journal of Rural Health, 30(4), 412–421. doi:10.1111/jrh.12070

Oser, C. B., Leukefeld, C. G., Cosentino-Boehm, A., & Havens, J. R. (2006). Rural HIV: Brief Interventions for felony probationers. American Journal of Criminal Justice: AJCJ, 31(1), 125–V.

Palamar, J. J., Shearston, J. A., Dawson, E. W., Mateu-Gelabert, P., & Ompad, D. C. (2016). Nonmedical opioid use and heroin use in a nationally representative sample of us high school seniors. Drug and Alcohol Dependence, 158, 132–138. doi:10.1016/j.drugalcdep.2015.11.005

Parker, J., Jackson, L., Dykeman, M., Gahagan, J., & Karabanow, J. (2012). Access to harm reduction services in Atlantic Canada: Implications for non-urban residents who inject drugs. Health and Place, 18(2), 152–162. doi:10.1016/j.healthplace.2011.08.016

Rosenblatt, R. A., Andrilla, C. H., Catlin, M., & Larson, E. H. (2015). Geographic and specialty distribution of US physicians trained to treat opioid use disorder. Annals of Family Medicine, 13(1), 23–26. doi:10.1370/afm.1735

Rosenblum, A., Cleland, C. M., Fong, C., Kayman, D., Tempalski, B., & Parrino, M. (2011). Distance traveled and cross-state commuting to opioid treatment programs in the United States. Journal of Environmental and Public Health, 2011, 1–10. doi:10.1155/2011/948789

Rosenblum, A., Parrino, M., Schnoll, S. H., Fong, C., Maxwell, C., Cleland, C. M., ... Haddox, J. D. (2007). Prescription opioid abuse among enrollees into methadone maintenance treatment. Drug and Alcohol Dependence, 90(1), 64–71. doi:10.1016/j.drugalcdep.2007.02.012

Rudavsky, S. (2016, April 11). An Indiana town recovering from 190 HIV cases. Indystar. Retrieved from http://www.indystar.com/story/news/2016/04/08/year-after-hiv-outbreak-austin-still-community-recovery/82133598/

Santa Ana, E. J., Stallings, D. L., Rounsaville, B. J., & Martino, S. (2013). Development of an in-home telehealth program for outpatient veterans with substance use disorders. Psychological Services, 10(3), 304–314. doi:10.1037/a0026511

Shannon, L. M., Havens, J. R., & Hays, L. (2010). Examining differences in substance use among rural and urban pregnant women. American Journal on Addictions, 19(6), 467–473. doi:10.1111/j.1521-0391.2010.00079.x

Sheehan, D. M., Trepka, M. J., Fennie, K. P., Prado, G., Madhivanan, P., Dillon, F. R., & Maddox, L. M. (2015). Individual and neighborhood predictors of mortality among HIV-positive Latinos with history of injection drug use, Florida, 2000–2011. Drug and Alcohol Dependence, 154, 243–250. doi:10.1016/j.drugalcdep.2015.07.007

Sorensen, J. L., & Copeland, A. L. (2000). Drug abuse treatment as an HIV prevention strategy: A review. *Drug and Alcohol Dependence, 59*(1), 17–31. doi:10.1016/S0376-8716(99)00104-0

Staton-Tindall, M., Harp, K. L., Minieri, A., Oser, C., Webster, J. M., Havens, J., & Leukefeld, C. (2015). An exploratory study of mental health and HIV risk behavior among drug-using rural women in jail. *Psychiatric Rehabilitation Journal, 38*(1), 45–54. doi:10.1037/prj0000107

Stein, B. D., Pacula, R. L., Gordon, A. J., Burns, R. M., Leslie, D. L., Sorbero, M. J., ... Dick, A. W. (2015). Where Is buprenorphine dispensed to treat opioid use disorders? The role of private offices, opioid treatment programs, and substance abuse treatment facilities in urban and rural counties. *Milbank Quarterly, 93*(3), 561–583. doi:10.1111/1468-0009.12137

Suryaprasad, A. G., White, J. Z., Xu, F., Eichler, B.-A., Hamilton, J., Patel, A., ... Holmberg, S. D. (2014). Emerging epidemic of hepatitis C virus infections among young nonurban persons who inject drugs in the United States, 2006–2012. *Clinical Infectious Diseases, 59*(10), 1411–1419. doi:10.1093/cid/ciu643

Sutton, M., Anthony, M. N., Vila, C., McLellan-Lemal, E., & Weidle, P. J. (2010). HIV testing and HIV/AIDS treatment services in rural counties in 10 southern states: Service provider perspectives. *Journal of Rural Health, 26*(3), 240–247. doi:10.1111/j.1748-0361.2010.00284.x

Tucker, J. A., Simpson, C. A., Huang, J., Roth, D. L., & Stewart, K. E. (2013). Utility of an interactive voice response system to assess antiretroviral pharmacotherapy adherence among substance users living with HIV/AIDS in the rural South. *AIDS Patient Care and STDS, 27*(5), 280–286. doi:10.1089/apc.2012.0322

van den Berg, C., Smit, C., van Brussel, G., Coutinho, R., & Prins, M. (2007). Full participation in harm reduction programmes is associated with decreased risk for human immunodeficiency virus and hepatitis C virus: Evidence from the Amsterdam cohort studies among drug users. *Addiction, 102*(9), 1454–1462. doi:10.1111/j.1360-0443.2007.01912.x

Van Handel, M. M., Rose, C. E., Hallisey, E. J., Kolling, J. L., Zibbell, J. E., Lewis, B., ... Brooks, J. T. (2016). County-level vulnerability assessment for rapid dissemination of HIV or HCV infections among persons who inject drugs, United States. *JAIDS Journal of Acquired Immune Deficiency Syndromes* (Publish ahead of print) doi:10.1097/qai.0000000000001098

Vestal, C. (2016). *An all-in response to the opioid crisis.* Retrieved from Washington, D.C. http://www.pewtrusts.org/en/research-and-analysis/blogs/stateline/2016/06/06/an-all-in-response-to-the-opioid-crisis

Vyavaharkar, M., Moneyham, L., Murdaugh, C., & Tavakoli, A. (2012). Factors associated with quality of life among rural women with HIV disease. *AIDS and Behavior, 16*(2), 295–303. doi:10.1007/s10461-011-9917-y

Wilson, L. E., Korthuis, T., Fleishman, J. A., Conviser, R., Lawrence, P. B., Moore, R. D., & Gebo, K. A. (2011). HIV-related medical service use by rural/urban residents: A multistate perspective. *AIDS Care, 23*(8), 971–979. doi:10.1080/09540121.2010.543878

Wood, S. A. (2008). Health care services for HIV-positive substance abusers in a rural setting: An innovative program. *Social Work in Health Care, 47*(2), 108–121. doi:10.1080/00981380801970202

Wright, P. B., Booth, B. M., Curran, G. M., Borders, T. F., Ounpraseuth, S. T., & Stewart, K. E. (2014). Correlates of HIV testing among rural African American cocaine users. *Research in Nursing and Health, 37*(6), 466–477. doi:10.1002/nur.21629

Wright, P. B., Stewart, K. E., Curran, G. M., & Booth, B. M. (2013). A qualitative study of barriers to the utilization of HIV testing services among rural African American cocaine users. *Journal of Drug Issues, 43*(3), 314–334. doi:10.1177/0022042613476260

Young, A. M., DiClemente, R. J., Halgin, D. S., Sterk, C. E., & Havens, J. R. (2014). HIV vaccine acceptability among high-risk drug users in Appalachia: A cross-sectional study. *BMC Public Health, 14,* 537. doi:10.1186/1471-2458-14-537

Young, A. M., Jonas, A. B., Mullins, U. L., Halgin, D. S., & Havens, J. R. (2013). Network structure and the risk for HIV transmission among rural drug users. *AIDS and Behavior, 17*(7), 2341–2351. doi:10.1007/s10461-012-0371-2

Ziller, E. C., Lenardson, J. D., & Coburn, A. F. (2012). Health care access and use among the rural uninsured. *Journal of Health Care for the Poor and Underserved, 23*(3), 1327–1345. doi:10.1353/hpu.2012.0100

Zukoski, A. P., & Thorburn, S. (2009). Experiences of stigma and discrimination among adults living with HIV in a low HIV-prevalence context: A qualitative analysis. *AIDS Patient Care and STDS, 23*(4), 267–276. doi:10.1089/apc.2008.0168

Zule, W. A., Costenbader, E., Coomes, C. M., Meyer, W. J., Jr., Riehman, K., Poehlman, J., & Wechsberg, W. M. (2007). Stimulant use and sexual risk behaviors for HIV in rural North Carolina. *Journal of Rural Health, 23*(Suppl), 73–78. doi:10.1111/j.1748-0361.2007.00127.x

Part III
Rural Families and Communities: Prevention and Intervention

Chapter 8
Our Experience: HIV-Positive African American Women in the Deep South

Catherine Wyatt-Morley

My Story

In March of 1994, my husband Tim, and I arrived at the hospital at 5:00 A.M. We were led to my room, where I was told to put on a hospital gown. Nervously changing, I got into bed as the nurse entered the room. She began going over the information I had provided a few days prior, then hung an IV and informed me that I would be moved soon. Tim stood bedside looking at me with loving eyes and gently kissed me. He whispered, "I love you," as I was wheeled beyond the double doors of pre-op.

Within hours of surgery, I was discharged to recuperate at home. The next morning I became ill. Tim rushed me to a nearby hospital where I was re-admitted, and my primary care doctor was notified. He told me the surgeon had discovered a problem with my blood before the surgery, and that I was discharged from the previous hospital too soon. He tried to reassure me that it was nothing serious, but his eyes said differently. The nurse came to draw my blood, but as she entered my room I noticed a Biohazard sign hanging on the outside of my door.

Days later, Tim drove me to the surgeon's office where I was immediately ushered into an exam room. The nurse, wearing plastic gloves, did not take my vitals; instead, she tossed a gown on the table and left the room. I lay in the paper gown, on the exam table, anticipating the surgeon's findings after his examination of me. The doctor entered the room, wearing plastic gloves, a surgical gown and

Catherine Wyatt-Morley in collaboration with Georgia Southern University.

C. Wyatt-Morley (✉)
Women On Maintaining Education and Nutrition, 417 Welshwood Drive, Suite 303, Nashville, TN 37211-4248, USA
e-mail: women@educatingwomen.org
URL: http://www.educatingwomen.org

facemask; he was eerily standoffish. As he stood across the room, not having touched me, he informed me that I was healing and admonished me to keep my appointment with the OB-GYN, set for 2:00 P.M. that day. I told him I was still in great pain, but he ignored my concerns. After dressing, I went to the front desk to pay the balance of my bill, but the office staff informed me the balance was forgiven, and I did not have to return. I left his office in pain, not understanding how he could say I was healing without doing a physical examination or addressing my pain.

Later that afternoon, seated in the crowded waiting room of my OB-GYN, the pain became excruciating. In response to my plea, Tim frantically informed the receptionist that we could no longer wait. The pain was just too unbearable. She rushed to inform the doctor, and we were hurriedly escorted to his office. Anxiety and worry gripped Tim as we quietly sat waiting for the doctor to enter the room. Still recovering from surgery, my body was weak, with blood penetrating through the bandages; I was miserable and aching with pain. My doctor, who has known Tim and me for years, solemnly told us that I had tested positive for the "Human Immunodeficiency Virus" (HIV), the virus that causes Acquired Immunodeficiency Syndrome (AIDS).

I was consumed with dread. His sledgehammer diagnosis exploded over me as fear suddenly took my imagination to all the images of AIDS, and the dark unknown. Bewildered, I asked the doctor, "Why was I tested? Who tested me?" He avoided my questions, focusing only on my wellbeing. I felt nauseated. The room began to spin as I told him he had to be mistaken. A long pause ensued as my life flashed before me. It was only supposed to be a simple hysterectomy, not HIV, not AIDS. I gasped for air, holding my pain-ridden stomach. I felt as if I were delivered into the hands of hell. How could this be? I was faithful to my husband. Immediately my thoughts shifted towards my three small children. Leaving my children motherless overwhelmed me. Resigned to the inevitable reality I would face, I asked, "What do we do now?" An unspoken stare between Tim and me was broken by Tim's words telling the doctor—he should also get tested. The doctor agreed and immediately contacted the adjoining hospital to make arrangements for Tim to be tested right away. As we left the office, walking slowly in silence, I wondered what had just happened. I sat in the car, waiting for Tim to have his blood drawn, and struggled to recall the doctor's words, realizing my life had instantly changed forever. Sitting alone, replaying recent events, I recalled my primary care doctor saying I had been discharged from the hospital too soon. Then it occurred to me, the surgeon had known. It became clear; the nurse not taking my vitals, the doctor not examining me, the Biohazard sign that hung outside my door, my medical bill balance forgiven—they all had known.

My first clinic appointment sucked. The waiting room was crowded, and it appeared no one wanted to make eye contact. Frequent emergencies occurred, so I waited. It was not like a regular doctor's office, at least not to me. I knew, as I looked around the room at the other people, they too were HIV-Positive or had AIDS. Some had small frames and could hardly walk, some looked healthy, and some were very sick. I saw different stages of myself in them. I had never even had a sexually transmitted disease (STD). Now, sitting in that waiting room, I became engulfed by the heaviness, the burden of having HIV. I took out my note pad and began writing another letter to my children. I detailed my love for each of them, the sadness they would endure upon their parents' deaths, and why the thought of leaving them was destroying me more than the disease. The next letter to them described our end of life requests. After being seated in one of the exam rooms, I began to compose myself. I asked lots of questions, and most were answered promptly in language I could understand. The nurse practitioner was very compassionate, taking time to listen to my concerns and questions. Tim's visit resulted in a prescription of Azidothymidine, better known as AZT, the dreaded monster drug—he was also HIV-Positive.

Healing slowly from the hysterectomy, my doctors suggested that before returning to work I see the company's medical director. I presented the physician with four letters from various medical providers and counselors, detailing my condition. After carefully reading the letters, his response was, "Go home, get your will made out, sell your house, and set up some place for your kids to live. There is nothing I can do to help you, not even temporarily." I informed him that he was the only person at the company who knew of my condition and that my doctors suggested I seek his help. His response was, "Don't worry. People will find out; you won't be able to keep this virus a secret. With all the sickness you got coming, you'll be lucky to have a job before it's over."

I begged him not to show those letters to anyone and not to keep them in my medical file. I even offered to take them back. "No, I better hold on to them," he said. He assured me no one would see the letters and that he would keep them "under lock and key." I could not believe his cruelty. I was shaking, crying, and totally hysterical by the time I left his office. Not wanting anyone to see me, I bolted out the door, ran to the car, and drove home in a daze. Talking with the medical director proved to be heartbreaking. Shortly thereafter, those letters, along with the content of my medical records, were copied and distributed throughout the company's workforce. Soon after, I began getting threatening phone calls.

As time passed, I became broken and bone-crushingly depressed. I felt hopeless, scared, and alone. Nothing seemed to console me, so I turned to my church, which had always brought me comfort. In the past, I had received the priest's guidance, prayers, and affirmation regarding our marital problems and believed I would now receive similar guidance. Trembling, I told him my husband and I had been diagnosed with HIV/AIDS, my experience with the surgeon, hospital, company doctor, and my fears for our family's future. He listened unmoved, offering nothing. The priest then told me I could no longer attend church services. I left without even an offered prayer. I left empty.

Reaching for support, I called my mother. Shocked, she wanted to know how this could happen. Composing herself, her questions turned to whether we had told anyone else in the family. She adamantly demanded I tell no one. Doing so would cause her embarrassment. Her words echoed in my ear, as her voice and presence drifted away from me. At that moment, I knew her support was gone.

Self-recrimination, anger, and frustration fueled Tim's rage as he withdrew to the bottom of a Vodka bottle, escaping our reality, as our marriage crumbled under the weight of HIV. I considered myself "safe" in a heterosexual, monogamous marriage. Like most Americans, I believed HIV/AIDS was in someone else's family, not a heterosexual, financially successful married couple. Not us! Not me! In a matter of weeks, I had been diagnosed HIV-Positive; my husband was diagnosed HIV-Positive, and he was immediately placed on the only available medication known at the time to treat HIV/AIDS.

Little did I know, I would lose everything: my job, health insurance, 401k, retirement benefits, car, church family, home, and friends; when I thought there was nothing else to lose, I was wrong. I lost weight, my confidence, my marriage, my mother's support, and, according to my prognosis, soon my life. With no appetite, no sleep, and no peace, my life became unrecognizable. Our dreams and plans for life were gone, but, through the veil of loss, heartache, and pain, a fire ignited. I wanted to fight for my life and my children's future, but the stress of HIV was immense and the depth of despair was dark, until I found a beacon of hope (Wyatt-Morley, 1997).

Making an Advocate

I was grateful when I met the phenomenal strength and encouragement I found in a beautiful, young African American HIV-Positive woman who became my beacon of hope, mentor, and sojourner. Born in the Mississippi Delta and living in Nashville, her abundant spirit was bottomless. Through her I began to see life as an HIV-Positive woman. Facing many challenges, including, at times, her very weak, skeletal-like frame being incrusted with lesions, she gave her time willingly and unconditionally, educating me about how to live life as an empowered HIV-Positive African American woman. Listening to her share the affronts of her suffering would have broken most; however, I was fortified to experience her herculean grace and sheer will power. She empowered me beyond comprehension; speaking words over me that I carry with me today. When she died in 1997, I was devastated.

Conversely, an activist was born. Educating myself became critical. I read articles, stories, the "Morbidity and Mortality Weekly Report," published by the Centers for Disease Control and Prevention (CDC), medical journals, papers, brochures, books, magazines, flyers, anything I could find, most of which pertained to HIV/AIDS in men. As I researched, I began to grasp the significance of being symptomatic vs. asymptomatic, viral loads, T-cell counts, T-8 ratios and opportunistic infections (OI). I also learned in 1981, that of the Centers for Disease Control and Prevention's (CDC) 26 reported cases of HIV, one was an African American (Gavett, 2012). That was significant news to me, because thirteen years later, HIV/AIDS had become very black and very female, as more and more cases, including mine, were revealed. I became consumed by the transforming influence of "ACT UP" New York, as their actions exploded across the media. I began attending national conferences in Washington DC, Philadelphia, and New York, where I met other HIV-Positive African American women. These conferences showed me the importance of gender-organizing, developing women-centered policies, planning, implementing meaningful demonstrations, and creating women-focused advocacy across the United States. I became electrified by the galvanized energy and power of those women.

Returning home, I was discontent. I began to prioritize strategies that focused on HIV-Positive African American women like me. Knowing one's status, as hard as it may be to accept, I believed, was important. As in my own case, treatment for women would be very different because family priorities would always take precedence, so resolving those stumbling blocks would mean more receptivity to treatment. The care received must be gender-centered; respectful of each woman's traditions and culture; acknowledging her experiences, concerns and opinions; providing services on her level of understanding; taking into consideration her personality, i.e., reserved, timid, scared, quiet or talkative; considering any history of abuse, substance use, and work and family life. If she is a mother, remaining mindful that her children would most likely come first.

These were important issues for me as an HIV-Positive wife and mother. So having secured an appointment, I was excited, as I eagerly entered the office of the director of the local AIDS service organization. Although I was armed with enthusiasm and a detailed plan, including ideas for developing women-centered services, addressing African American cultural nuances, engaging the African American church, combating stigma, and ways to empower local women, my plan was rejected. My ideas were dismissed as inadequate. I was taken aback, as the agency director spoke condescendingly, laughing me out of his office. Before this encounter, I believed everyone in my community who was HIV-Positive cared and wanted everyone who was HIV-Positive to have the best services available in our community. Disillusioned, I learned early that I was not the right gender or the right color, and was therefore not welcome at certain local policy tables. My experiences as a heterosexual African American woman and mother living with HIV in the South did not fit in with the *good ole boy* infrastructure. Women, specifically black women, had their place, but I continually, purposefully, refused to stay in my place.

Naively, I unexpectedly entered into a well-oiled political network of backdoor deals, favoritism, and close ties, which were obviously established for mutual benefit. My opinions regarding the needs of HIV-Positive African American women were devalued, dismissed as irrelevant to the local agenda. Kept out of the loop for meetings regarding funding, and strategies, I had an opinion and expressed it, loudly. I pushed back using the media when I did not agree, which was often, since resources for HIV-Positive women, specifically HIV-Positive African American women's needs were going unaddressed. Although my type of advocacy was unwelcomed, my heart was heavily burdened with loss, stigma, discrimination, rejection, and the mistreatment I had endured. I was determined to fulfill the promise I had made to my sojourner, to become an advocate.

So, where there was no voice for African American women living with HIV/AIDS in my community, I became that voice. Where there was no women-centered HIV/AIDS programming, I created it. Where there was no women-centered support group, I formed one. Where there was no food pantry to meet the needs of African American women living with HIV/AIDS, I organized one. Where there were no massage therapy, holistic care, and nutrition services, that met the needs of African American women living with HIV/AIDS, I produced them.

Advocacy included becoming a member of the Tennessee State HIV/AIDS Prevention Community Planning Group led by a regal African American woman. I also became a member of the Ryan White Community AIDS Partnership well before Ryan White funding came to Tennessee. Nationally, I became a member of the National Minority AIDS Council and the National Association of People with AIDS. I garnered six television, radio, and newspaper interviews, all by 1995.

My focus became women of color, gender disparities, reproductive health, and heterosexual transmission of HIV. I recognized immediately that heterosexual transmission was an important aspect of the epidemic for African American women, since heterosexual transmission, by far, was the most common mode of HIV transmission among African American women in the United States and the South.

Determined not to die from a misunderstood disease, I read, became a member of additional national HIV/AIDS organizations, made lots of gay and straight HIV-Positive friends, met advocates, listened intently on national conference calls, and prayed, as my home crumbled. With my marriage in ruins, and my children always in the forefront of my every thought, my letters to them intensified, recognizing their trauma and the sorrow HIV/AIDS was yet to bring them. The letters to my children, since the first day of my diagnosis, kept me sane in the insanity of HIV.

With my children's encouragement, and to the disgrace of my mother, I began speaking publicly. The video I produced, *Reasons to Live; Women Their Families and HIV,* premiered at Vanderbilt Scarritt Bennett Center in 1996 to a packed audience, and my book, *AIDS Memoir: Journal of an HIV Positive Mother,* taken from the letters written to my children, was published in 1997. I was accepted as a member of the Adult AIDS Clinical Trial Group; Community Constituency Group, (ACTG/CCG), where I served on the Patient Care Committee for five years. The ACTG/CCG taught me the structure and science of HIV/AIDS research and the importance of data-driven advocacy. Accepting an invitation to Mountain House, in Caux, Switzerland, in 1998, I became the first HIV-Positive African American woman to open discussions on the worldwide HIV pandemic among women and girls.

Disgraceful Disease

By definition the word *stigma* means "mark of disgrace." A powerful word, stigma has transformed attitudes about HIV/AIDS into a negative social phenomenon. HIV-related stigma remains one of the greatest barriers to the health and wellbeing of HIV-Positive African American women. As people were dying daily, stigma remained entrenched into the very fabric of the disease. I began seeing several factors emerge.

First, the way the media portrayed HIV/AIDS seemed censored and different from my reality. Second, although several modes of transmission have been identified, HIV was shrouded in the evils of sex, especially in the South. There was a culture of silence that surrounded sex, dictating that "good" women are expected to be passive, even subservient, and submissive. Third, women's economic dependency amplified their HIV susceptibility, making them more likely to remain in an abusive relationship (Kaiser Family Foundation, 2013, 2014a, b). Women, for a variety of reasons, were most often not able to negotiate condom use. I watched as gender inequality, stigma, and discrimination kept HIV-Positive African American women quiet, suppressing their painful experiences (Editorial, 2006). Fourth, the rate of African American male incarceration was increasing dramatically, as the drug scene was amplified and linked to HIV (Adimora & Harawa, 2008; Johnson & Raphael, 2005; El-Sadr, Mayer, & Adimora, 2010). Fifth, how a person became infected mattered: those who became infected through drug use or homosexuality were treated differently than those who were born infected, were babies infected from breast milk, or were "innocently" infected heterosexually. The latter evoked sympathy, the former evoked harsh judgment (Herek, 2003).

The early days of HIV/AIDS set profound indicators of disease trends, which affect today's economy, employment, housing, family dynamics, self-worth, treatment, and care for HIV-Positive African American women (National Rural Health Association, 2014). Stigma, shame, blame, and denial became embedded in the American psyche, especially in African American culture, bringing with it deadly consequences.

As the pandemic continued to outpace efforts to control it, the number of newly infected African American women steadily outnumbered those who gained access to treatment. Disease misconception caused widespread persistent and pervasive stigma, leaving in its wake isolation, depression, self-loathing, rejection, violence, separation, abandonment, suicide, and broken families; thus, becoming a serious impediment for accessing HIV testing, prevention, care, and treatment services.

Distrust of the government stemming from the Tuskegee Syphilis experiment remains salient to significant numbers of rural African Americans in the South (Brandt, 1978; W.O.M.E.N., 2016). This multi-generational mistrust is difficult to change as scores of African Americans, in general, believe "the government is using AIDS to kill off minority groups" (Manuel-Logan, 2012). In the Deep South, conspiracy beliefs continue to impede access to HIV care, treatment, and medication adherence.

Women On Maintaining Education and Nutrition

In 1994, shortly after I was diagnosed, I established Women On Maintaining Education and Nutrition, W.O.M.E.N., because there were no HIV/AIDS services designed specifically for heterosexual HIV-Positive African American women like me in my community. What started as a small support group, named "Women On

Reasons To Heal," (W.O.R.T.H.) in a bedroom of my home became a safe space for women, mothers, and families impacted by HIV/AIDS to find camaraderie and encouragement through difficult times while also celebrating each of life's joys. I found the supportive relationships with other HIV-Positive women offered constant learning, words of wisdom, experiences, and hope. The indestructible bond of sisterhood was present each time one of us entered the hospital, and each time one of us died. Led by HIV-Positive women for HIV-Positive women, W.O.R.T.H.'s membership grew, as women from as far away as Paducah, Kentucky and Birmingham, Alabama attended. Emboldened and empowered, we found caring and life-giving strength in one another.

Today, W.O.M.E.N. serves a highly diverse group of HIV-Positive African American and other minority women across the HIV care continuum and the socioeconomic spectrum. Our program participants also include women who have experienced Post Traumatic Stress Disorder and Lesbian, Bisexual and Transgender (LBT) women. What most of our women share in common is their fear of HIV status exposure and the lack of available mental health and social support.

Following years of discussion, collecting data from questionnaires, surveys, opinion polls and seeking the input of HIV-Positive African American women around the country, W.O.M.E.N strives to eliminate antiquated care, making dramatic changes that embody comprehensive, multidimensional, culturally compassionate care models that integrate physical, emotional, mental and spiritual wholeness to meet the unique, complex, diverse and essential needs of HIV-Positive women. As an African American woman living with AIDS, I believe that a twenty-first century individualized mind, body, spirit agenda, centering on increased self-esteem, self-care, self-worth, and interpersonal skills, empowers women in their HIV education, care, and treatment. This can only happen in a nonjudgmental atmosphere of safety, respect and acceptance.

HIV-Positive African American Women in the Deep South

The following are some of the shared perspectives of 32 HIV-Positive African American women, between the ages of 20 and 65, residing in the Deep South. Collectively and individually, the group provides observations and examples of how HIV-related stigma continues to permeate African American communities in the Deep South, hindering prevention, testing, and treatment.

United in our belief, "That too many of us living with HIV/AIDS in the Deep South are desperately poor, do not receive gender-specific HIV education, struggle to survive, and shelter in urban and rural decay. Several of us have incomes less than $10,000 per year, live in extremely rural areas far from treatment facilities, and experience unstable housing which often leads to homelessness. We are, at times, forced into unprotected survival sex, raise children in drug infested environments, inhabit deplorable unsanitary conditions, depend on others for transportation, and experience serious medical service barriers."

Rasheda stated, "As an African American woman I give my all in a relationship. I look for a faithful relationship, and I have to have condom-less intercourse 'cause he keeps a roof over my children's heads, pays the bills, and puts food on the table. Cause if I mention protection, he'll hit, quit, or split."

The previously mentioned 32 African American women living with HIV/AIDS in the Deep South agree that, "Money drives everything!" Considering the history of the Deep South, current HIV statistics, and the urgent need to address HIV disparities, Sabrina, one of the 32 women asks, "Why is funding not where it should be? For as long as HIV/AIDS has existed in the United States, why are all of us still not able to access lifesaving services? Why in the Deep South, are many of us turned away, made to feel 'less than', suffer reproductive injustice, and not provided the information or support needed to make healthy choices for ourselves and our children? Why are black children in the Deep South growing up motherless because their mother died of AIDS, when AIDS is now treated as a chronic disease?"

To further the discussion, the group agreed that, "Many African American women living with HIV/AIDS in the Deep South raise their children without fathers in the home." LaTonya said, "When we die, our black children act out, become truant teens, or become black men in jail. If African American women are heterosexually disproportionately infected and dying, why is the money not supporting the epidemiology? When the objective of HIV funding is to strengthen support, expand prevention responses, provide linkage, navigation, and supportive care, reduce individual and community HIV/AIDS vulnerability, and alleviate the impact of the epidemic, why then, are current women-focused, women-service organizations in the Deep South, which have demonstrated records of serving African American women living with HIV/AIDS, going under funded or without funding? Most organizations here in the Deep South are currently not funded to provide women-centered HIV services. Most do not provide peer based women's support groups. Am I greater than AIDS or is AIDS greater than me? Does my life actually matter? Or am I disposable?"

Group member, Tamera said, "Rural or urban, my HIV-Positive Deep South experience overwhelmingly sees the epidemic as poor, black, brown, mocha, almond and female. More money is sent by the United States to third world countries than is spent at home for African American women living with HIV/AIDS in the Deep South. Why is that?"

As American women living with HIV/AIDS in the Deep South, we wonder, "Do black lives really matter? How can black lives matter when the givers of black life, living in perpetual, deplorable, debilitating conditions, experience such perplexing lack?" One member stated, "Black lives cannot matter without black women giving birth to those black lives."

Another cultural complication for HIV-Positive African American women in the Deep South is gossip. As Cassandra said, "Scandal spreads in small rural communities when your doctor lives around the corner, the lady looking at your medical records lives across the street, the nurse taking your vitals lives up the block, a next-door neighbor works at the health department, and your family works at the clinic." Gossip becomes commonplace as people thrive on the hardships of others, which in turn drives African American women away from treatment and the healthcare system. Cassandra also added, "HIPAA does not exist when people talk to people, confidentiality is breached, accountability does not apply, and our anonymity becomes community scandal."

Developing Solutions

Call to Action

Over the course of the twenty-three years since my diagnosis, many treatment advances have occurred. However, African American women living with HIV/AIDS in the Deep South remain grossly underrepresented in decision making AIDS institutions, funding allocations, community planning, boards of directors, and executive positions. These women have creative ideas, untapped wisdom, unique perspectives, and possess the ability to make meaningful contributions to the disparities in our communities. Such intelligence is essential in highlighting the HIV-Positive African American woman's Deep South experience. Unanimously, the 32 HIV-Positive African American women believe there is an urgent need for modernized innovative high-quality care, strengthening unification and forward-thinking, gender-centered education and recommend the following course of action.

Vital is the development of a one body, nine member oversight "Brain-Trust." The HIV-Positive African American women living in the Deep South, first of its kind Brain-Trust, will be created by HIV-Positive African American women living in the Deep South who will identify and solve problems, using their extensive experience and knowledge. Facilitated by the founder of W.O.M.E.N., each woman will represent one of the denoted nine Deep South states. They will create a hallmark of health within the HIV African American community. The Brain-Trust will identify specific prevention treatment and care protocols, create new opportunities to collaborate, create networks that serve underserved communities, link our collective to other networks, connect to and establish relationships with national leaders, unify our common vision, and develop culturally specific data and research. The Brain-Trust will partner with: universities and institutions of higher education; government officials; hospitals, doctor's offices, pharmacies, libraries and community centers, volunteers, interns; HIV and non-HIV community-based organizations, and community health clinics; pharmaceutical companies; businesses, philanthropists; churches, mom and pop shops, gatekeepers; mental health providers; IT and the media.

The *Call To Action*, illustrates the readiness of HIV-Positive African American women to collaboratively contribute to an inclusive robust agenda which addresses the vital disparities in the nine Deep South states. African American women living with HIV/AIDS in the South have the innate capacity to actively participate in meaningful, respectful intergenerational conversations, planning and service implementation which reflects our challenges, experiences, and resiliency.

I earnestly take this opportunity to convey my deepest appreciation and heartfelt gratitude for the kindness of the brave women who shared their thoughts, ideas, experiences, challenges, and tears, as I formulated this chapter. For future information regarding W.O.M.E.N., chapter author, chapter content, to become a supporter, partner, or to get involved, please contact the author.

References

About Us. (2016). *Women On Maintaining Education and Nutrition*. Retrieved from http://www.educatingwomen.org/about-us/

Adimora, A., & Harawa, N. (2008). Incarceration, African Americans, and HIV: Advancing a research agenda. *Journal of the National Medical Association, 100*(1). 57–62. doi:10.1016/S0027-9684(15)31175-5

Brandt, A. M. (1978, December). The case of the Tuskegee Syphilis study. *Hastings Center Magazine*. Retrieved from http://www.med.navy.mil/bumed/Documents/Healthcare%20Ethics/Racism-And-Research.pdf

El-Sadr, W. M., Mayer, K. H., & Adimora, A. A. (2010). The HIV epidemic in the United States a time for action. *Journal of Acquired Immune Deficiency Syndrome, 55*(2), 63–67. Retrieved from http://journals.lww.com/SiteCollectionDocuments/DM/JAIDS_12152010_Supplement.pdf

Gavett, G. (2012, July). *Timeline: 30 years of AIDS in Black America*. Retrieved from http://www.pbs.org/wgbh/frontline/article/timeline-30-years-of-aids-in-black-america/#81

Herek, G. M. (2003). HIV/AIDS Stigma and the General Population. Resource Center: *The body*. Retrieved from http://www.thebody.com/content/art12405.html

Johnson, R. C., & Raphael, S. (2005, July). *Effects of male incarceration dynamics on AIDS infection rates among African-American women and men*. Unpublished manuscript, Goldman School of Public Policy, University of California, Berkley, California. Retrieved from https://www.law.yale.edu/system/files/documents/pdf/The_Effects_of_Male_Incarceration_Dynamics.pdf

Kaiser Family Foundation. (2013, April). *A report on women and HIV/AIDS in the U.S.* Retrieved from https://kaiserfamilyfoundation.files.wordpress.com/2013/04/8436.pdf

Kaiser Family Foundation. (2014a, March). *Women and HIV/AIDS in the United States*. Retrieved from http://kff.org/hivaids/fact-sheet/women-and-hivaids-in-the-united-states/

Kaiser Family Foundation. (2014b, March). *Women and HIV/AIDS in the United States*. Retrieved from https://kaiserfamilyfoundation.files.wordpress.com/2014/03/6092-women-and-hivaids-in-the-united-states1.pdf

Manuel-Logan, R. (2012). *Black conspiracy theories 101: HIV/AIDS was created to extinguish blacks [Web log post]*. Retrieved from http://newsone.com/2026978/black-urban-legends-hiv-aids/

National Rural Health Association. (2014, April). *HIV/AIDS in rural America: Disproportionate impact on minority and multicultural populations* (Policy Brief). Retrieved from https://www.ruralhealthweb.org/getattachment/Advocate/Policy-Documents/HIVAIDSRuralAmericapolicybriefApril2014-%281%29.pdf.aspx?lang=en-US

Stigma, Discrimination and HIV. (n.d.). *AVERT*. Retrieved from http://www.avert.org/professionals/hiv-social-issues/stigma-discrimination

Wyatt-Morley, C. (1997). *AIDS Memoir: Journal of an HIV-Positive Mother*. West Hartford, Connecticut: Kumarian Press Inc.

Chapter 9
Intersecting HIV Prevention Practice and Truth Among Black MSM

Stacy W. Smallwood, Jarvis W. Carter Jr. and Anne O. Odusanya

Introduction

In June 2010, President Barack Obama decreed the following:

> The United States will become a place where new HIV infections are rare and when they do occur, every person, regardless of age, gender, race/ethnicity, sexual orientation, gender identity or socio-economic circumstance, will have unfettered access to high-quality, life-extending care, free from stigma and discrimination ("National HIV/AIDS Strategy for the United States," 2010).

Since his announcement, the nation has witnessed a reduction in new HIV infections for some populations, but increases in others, particularly among young Black men who have sex with men (MSM) ages 13–34 years (CDC, 2015b) and primarily among those living in the U.S. South (CDC, 2016a; Reif et al., 2014, 2015). Today, there are approximately 1.2 million people living with HIV in the United States (CDC, 2015a, b), of which MSM accounted for 67% of new HIV infections in 2014, with 38% and 26% of those new infections being attributed to Black or African American (hereafter referred to as Black) and Hispanic MSM,

S.W. Smallwood (✉)
Department of Community Health Behavior & Education, Jiann-Ping Hsu College of Public Health, Georgia Southern University, 501 Forest Drive, P.O. Box 8015 Statesboro, GA 30460, USA
e-mail: ssmallwood@georgiasouthern.edu

J.W. Carter Jr.
Division of HIV/AIDS Prevention/Prevention Research Branch, Centers for Disease Control & Prevention, 1600 Clifton Road, NE Mailstop: E-37, Atlanta, GA 30329, USA
e-mail: JWCarter@cdc.gov

A.O. Odusanya
Department of Community Health Behavior and Education, Jiann-Ping Hsu College of Public Health, Georgia Southern University, 501 Forest Drive, Statesboro, GA 30460, USA
e-mail: ao01531@georgiasouthern.edu

© Springer International Publishing AG 2017
F.M. Parks et al. (eds.), *HIV/AIDS in Rural Communities*,
DOI 10.1007/978-3-319-56239-1_9

respectively (CDC, 2015b). These data exemplify the continuing HIV disparity among these diverse populations of men in comparison to other racial/ethnic MSM.

Thirty plus years into the HIV epidemic in this country, we now have an array of HIV prevention tools in our repertoire. Traditional HIV prevention methods for MSM focused on individual-level behavior modifications such as increased condom use and distribution of clean injection drug equipment (Fisher & Smith, 2009; Kennedy & Fonner, 2014). Contemporary HIV prevention tools saw biomedical advancements through the introduction of highly active antiretroviral treatment (HAART) in the mid-1990s, which substantially improved the quality of life for HIV-positive individuals (CDC, 2016b; National Institute on Drug Abuse, 2012). More recently, pre-exposure prophylaxis (PrEP) through the use of Truvada® (CDC, 2014a, b; Grant et al., 2010) is another biomedical HIV prevention option for populations disproportionately impacted by HIV such as Black MSM, but more generally for HIV-negative individuals at high risk for HIV infection as part of a comprehensive HIV prevention plan. The new biomedical approaches complement the individual-level methods of HIV prevention; however, we still continue to see Black MSM being impacted heavily by HIV. With the advent of the National HIV/AIDS Strategy (NHAS), the nation was charged with providing a more coordinated national response to HIV in the U.S.

One of the leading HIV prevention agencies in the country, the Centers for Disease Control and Prevention (CDC), was heavily influenced by the NHAS, which led to the high-impact prevention (HIP) strategy (CDC, 2011). HIP seeks to scale up the most cost-effective and scientifically based HIV prevention interventions such as targeted HIV testing toward populations impacted most by HIV, particularly communities of color, condom distribution programs, and biomedical approaches such as treatment as prevention for HIV-positive and HIV-negative individuals through antiretroviral treatment (ART) and PrEP, respectively. Some prevention strategies have demonstrated effectiveness in increasing HIV testing and engagement in HIV care for some populations; however, the HIV disparity among Black MSM continues to persist. Given the increase in new HIV infections among young Black MSM, particularly young Black MSM in the U.S. South, novel intervention methods and frameworks are needed to augment the achievements of the aforementioned HIV prevention methods.

Research has shown that Black MSM are as likely or less likely to engage in sexual risk behaviors associated with HIV when compared to White MSM (Millett, Flores, Peterson, & Bakeman, 2007a, 2012); however, the literature indicates that Black MSM are more likely to be diagnosed with a sexually transmitted disease, have a late diagnosis of HIV, and are less likely to be engaged in HIV medical care and be virally suppressed (Millett et al. 2007a). These latter dispositions have serious implications for engaging Black MSM along the HIV continuum of care (from HIV diagnosis to viral suppression of HIV). If individually linked behaviors such as engagement in condomless anal intercourse (CAI)[1] do not explain the HIV disparity within this population, what other factors beyond the aforementioned contribute to this gap? Furthermore, how do we lessen the HIV disparity among Black MSM?

HIV prevention scientists have long advocated for the need to focus more on social, structural, and contextual factors in research and practice to provide more insight on potential contributors to HIV infection among these men (Mays, Cochran, & Zamudio, 2004; Millett, Malcbranche, & Peterson, 2007b; Peterson & Jones, 2009). As one of the NHAS' goals emphasizes "reducing HIV-related disparities," this provides an opportunity for researchers, health professionals, and practitioners to explore and address social and structural factors contributing to the HIV disparity among Black MSM, but again, how do we tackle such an arduous task? One approach is to gain a better understanding of the experiences unique to Black MSM that hinder or facilitate them from receiving the quality care needed after HIV diagnosis or with obtaining an HIV test.

While recent data indicate that attitudes toward gay, bisexual, and other MSM (collectively referred to as MSM) are more favorable now than in the past (Glick & Golden, 2010), there are still persisting negative attitudes and challenges Black MSM encounter due to HIV-related stigma, racial discrimination, gender-role expectation expressions, and other prejudices (Dowshen, Binns, & Garofalo, 2009; Fullilove, West, Wilson, & Wright, 1997; Lemelle and Battle 2004; Lewis 2003; Vincent, Peterson, & Parrott, 2009). For Black MSM, living in the ever-present context of these societal challenges leads them to view and experience the world from a unique standpoint that can be regarded as their "truth" (Harding, 2004). If the lived experiences constitute truth for Black MSM, what does that truth look like? The truth for Black MSM is that they embody multiple socially-constructed identities that collectively shape their human existence. The truth of these men influences the degree to which they are accepted, understood, and appreciated by their families, friends, institutions, and society at-large. To understand the truth of Black MSM is to look beyond their singular identities (e.g., being Black only or MSM only), but rather to fully recognize the complexities of their experiences when their multiple identities converge. In the context of HIV prevention, it is important for public health professionals and clinical practitioners to be cognizant of the contextual factors that can influence health outcomes of Black MSM.

In an example of a Black MSM who experiences dual effects of discrimination from society and family, his race and sexuality are important factors to consider when he is seeking treatment or trying to identify a culturally appropriate venue to visit for HIV testing, but there are other considerations as well. Does this Black MSM live in a rural area where transportation resources may be scarce or in a close-knit community where confidentiality concerns may arise? Does this

---

[1]The term condomless anal intercourse (CAI) is used instead of the more traditionally used term unprotected anal intercourse (UAI) to use more precise language based on modern HIV prevention strategy advances (e.g., pre-exposure prophylaxis or antiretroviral treatment).

Black MSM have formal education or sufficient income to not only provide for his day-to-day needs, but for his HIV medications whether he is HIV positive or negative? The questions posed here can lay the foundation for this individual to gain access to HIV testing or care, and also receive a higher standard of care as he navigates through a sometimes intricate health care and social services system. Understanding the various ways in which different components of an individual's life converge and diverge gives breadth and depth to the framework of intersectionality, which is described in detail below.

In the remaining sections of this chapter, we provide an overview of the intersectionality framework along with pertinent theories, empirical evidence demonstrating the use of intersectionality in research and practice, and offer dialogue on future directions for HIV prevention among Black MSM, particularly those in the Southern U.S.

What Is Intersectionality?

Using intersectional frameworks in research methodology and practice could be one of the missing links to effectively reduce HIV among marginalized communities. The framework offers a thorough understanding and appreciation for a person's lived experiences and can offer insight as to what strategies may be useful or detrimental to really creating a United States where new HIV infections are rare. As we collectively strive to achieve the goals of NHAS, it is imperative to remain mindful that while important, HIV is not a priority for many of the marginalized communities we seek to serve. Incorporating intersectional frameworks into our HIV prevention methods, practices, and interventions can serve to mitigate the HIV disparity among Black MSM through coordinated efforts to address their entire truth.

Intersectionality is a theoretical framework that examines how multiple socially-constructed identities intersect at the micro-level of individual experience to expose multiple structural, macro-level inequalities (Crenshaw, 1989, 1991; Weber, 2010). Although its roots are in legal studies, intersectionality is becoming more widely recognized as a valuable tool in public health research and practice (Bowleg, 2012). Here, we will describe the basic tenets and origins of intersectionality and explain how it can be applied to HIV prevention practice for Black MSM.

Intersectionality begins with the recognition that individuals have multiple socially-constructed identities. People use many markers to define identities—race, gender, sexual orientation, socioeconomic class, geographic location, religion, and ability (e.g., being able-bodied or not able-bodied) are just some examples used to describe a person's identity and social location. Within each of those identity markers, there are groups that are socially privileged (advantaged) and those that are socially oppressed (discriminated against or disadvantaged). For example, in the

United States, a White racial identity is often associated with privilege, while many people of color experience significant disadvantages and discrimination based on their racial identity (Harawa & Ford, 2009; Jones, 2000). Similarly, men often have gender privileges, while women and gender-non-conforming people are disadvantaged.

While each social identity category contains groups that are privileged and groups that are not privileged, people belong to many different social groups and can experience privilege and oppression simultaneously. For example, a Black MSM may experience privilege related to his gender identity, while also being discriminated against or stigmatized for his racial and sexual identities. Intersectionality, then, helps us to see how a person's multiple identities intersect to reveal the "different types of discrimination and disadvantage that occur as a consequence of the combination of identities" (Association for Women's Rights in Development 2004, p. 2). By recognizing the complexities of an individual's multiple intersecting identities, we can gain a deeper understanding of how experiences with different types of discrimination and privilege impact HIV-related outcomes for Black MSM.

Origins of Intersectionality

Intersectionality as a theoretical framework originated in legal studies and is rooted in anti-racism work (Bauer, 2014), deriving from a Black feminist critique of the ways in which race and gender were treated as "mutually exclusive categories of experience and analysis" (Crenshaw, 1989, p. 139). Noted legal scholar Crenshaw (1989, 1991) used intersectionality to examine the experiences of Black women in the courts, and how their claims of racial and sexual discrimination were not understood or recognized as valid. Crenshaw used the 1977 court case *DeGraffenreid v. General Motors* to illustrate this point. In this case, five Black women sued General Motors (GM), claiming that GM's seniority system was discriminatory against Black women. The courts, however, ruled in favor of GM, stating that the plaintiffs could not make a claim based *only* on sex discrimination (since GM had White women as clerical employees), nor could their claim be based only on race discrimination (since GM hired Black men as manufacturing employees). Because of the court's lack of acknowledgment for the intersection of racial and sexual identities, the claims of discrimination were not recognized. Crenshaw (1991) later expanded the application of intersectionality to cases of violence against women, and how the experiences of women of color were not represented in feminist or anti-racist discourse. Although intersectionality began in legal studies, it has been utilized in many other areas, including political science, psychology, sociology, public health, social work, women's and gender studies, and human rights (Bowleg, 2012; Cole, 2009; Rasmussen, 2014).

Evolution of Intersectionality

Other scholars have used intersectionality in research, practice, and analytical approaches to fill in gaps or offer more concrete evidence of people's lived experiences. In her book, Understanding Race, Class, Gender, and Sexuality: A Conceptual Framework, Weber (2010) expands upon the foundation laid by Crenshaw by examining each of the core principles of an intersectionality framework and providing case study examples of how to apply this lens to collected data or even how to frame intersectionality questions. Weber also posits that, when analyzing intersecting identities such as race, class, gender, and sexuality, it is important to remain cognizant of the core principles that these identities (1) are historically and geographically contextual; (2) are socially-constructed; (3) are entwined with power relations; (4) operate at both the macro-level structural (institutional) and micro-level (individual); and (5) are simultaneously expressed.

As previously mentioned, intersectionality is a multi-disciplinary framework that has relevance in public health work as well. Bowleg (2012) identifies three major tenets of intersectionality. First, social identities are not independent, but are interconnected, and each social identity is informed and shaped by the experience of the other identities (Dottolo & Stewart, 2008). Second, individuals from identity groups that have been historically oppressed or marginalized should be the starting point for understanding disparate health outcomes (Bowleg, 2012). Third, the intersection of an individual's multiple identities can help us to identify larger level social and structural inequities (Bowleg, 2013).

Intersectionality as a framework helps us to see the experiences and oppressions faced by members of marginalized groups. How, though, do these experiences of discrimination and oppression affect health? Research suggests that members of marginalized groups are subjected to chronic stress related to their minority identities. Long-term exposure to this chronic stress has been associated with disparities in physical and mental health outcomes among oppressed groups, including substance abuse, anxiety, depression, and suicidality (DiPlacido, 1998; Hatzenbuehler, 2009; Mays & Cochran, 2001; Meyer, 1995; Williams & Mohammed, 2009). Therefore, it is important to examine other pertinent theories and models that may be used in conjunction with an intersectional approach.

The minority stress theory, first posited by Meyer (1995, 2003), suggests that the stress associated with a minority identity (such as a sexual minority identity) can lead to adverse mental health outcomes. The stresses associated with minority identity result, in part, from dissonance between the minority person's identity and the prevailing negative attitudes toward minority identities among the dominant culture. These negative attitudes often become internalized and manifest as adverse mental health outcomes and psychological distress (Dentato, 2012; Krieger et al., 2008; Meyer, 1995). However, minority stressors can also directly impact biological stress mechanisms (Friedman, Williams, Singer, & Ryff, 2009), affect engagement in health behaviors (Krieger et al., 2008), or influence the use of health services (Cochran, Sullivan, & Mays, 2003).

The tenets of intersectionality, coupled with minority stress theory, are especially salient for understanding the lived experiences of Black MSM, especially those living in the U.S. South. Jones, Wilton, Millett, and Johnson (2010) formulated the Stress and Severity Model of Minority Stress (SMS) for Black MSM, which is a model that focuses on stressors due to a person being a racial and sexual minority. The SMS model expands upon Meyer's minority stress model in that it accounts for other minority stressors beyond sexual identity. As such, it is imperative for public health practitioners and researchers to understand that there are differences in the social stressors that a Black MSM experiences in comparison to a White MSM. In either case, the SMS and minority stress theory are examples of existing theories that may be supplemented by intersectional approaches or analyses especially for Black MSM.

The truth for many Black MSM is that their existence intersects at being Black, male, and MSM—each of which carries its own unique characteristics and oppressions, but becomes something more than the sum of its parts when they manifest together in the same body. Central to that experience are the multiple historical oppressions that have been imposed upon Black people generally, Black males in particular, and sexual minority people in the U.S. Finally, the individual experiences of Black MSM in the rural South are framed by social climates (e.g., perceptions of Black male masculinity, acceptability of homosexuality in Black and rural communities) and institutional policies and practices (e.g., religious doctrinal opposition to the morality of homosexuality). In order to develop effective strategies to improve the health and well-being of Black MSM in these areas, it is important to examine these sociocultural and institutional effects through the intersectional lens of Black MSM's lived experiences.

Intersectionality, HIV, and Black MSM

Intersectionality can be a vital tool for the development and implementation of successful, evidence-based HIV prevention interventions (Bowleg, 2012; Wilson et al., 2015). Research suggests that addressing the various types of stigma that Black MSM encounter is an important component of culturally competent interventions. However, there is a scarcity of studies that employ an intersectional framework among Black MSM in their research design (Beatty, Wheeler, & Gaiter, 2004; Bowleg, 2012).

In a systematic review conducted by Wilson et al. (2015), stigma was intertwined with multiple identities among Black MSM pertaining to race, ethnicity, sexual orientation, social class, and gender along with HIV status. The majority of qualitative studies included in the systematic review emphasized that the numerous forms of identity-based stigma experienced by Black MSM were associated with increased HIV infection risk (Wilson et al., 2015). Multiple types of identity-based stigma can also result in poor health outcomes stemming from reduced access to comprehensive and culturally competent HIV prevention and care services (Haile, Padilla, &

Parker, 2011; Miller, Serner, & Wagner, 2005). To further demonstrate some of the barriers Black MSM encounter, evidence shows that institutional stigma and stereotypes concerning Black men can negatively impact them by reducing their chances of obtaining employment and receiving substance use treatment, ultimately exacerbating HIV risk behaviors (Tobin, Cutchin, Latkin, & Takahashi, 2013). Data from national-level surveys further highlight economic disparities in that Black men in same-sex couples were more than six times as likely to live in poverty as their White counterparts (Badgett, Durso, & Schneebaum, 2013). There is a litany of external challenges that Black MSM must cope with due to heterosexism, homophobia, classism, and racism (Bowleg, Teti, Malebranche, & Tschann, 2013; Parker and Aggleton, 2003). Depending upon the circumstances, some Black MSM cope better than others. To that point, use of an intersectional framework lends itself to identifying, understanding, and addressing the day-to-day nuances in the lived experiences of Black MSM. This framework could have a drastic impact on reducing the HIV disparity among this group of men by adequately tackling the social and institutional inequities currently plaguing many of their lives in the Southern U.S.

In intersectional frameworks, identities are not simply additive, but more multiplicative; when individual identities intersect, they create something unique, in which the experience of one social identity cannot be fully understood without recognizing the other interlocking social identities (Bowleg, 2012). In previous qualitative research, Black MSM have expressed that they experience difficulty separating their identities of race, gender, sexual identity and more; for example, Black MSM have found it difficult to articulate their experiences as men without viewing those experiences through the racial lens of being a Black man, and in some cases, through both a racial *and* sexual lens of being a Black gay man (Bowleg, 2012). The Black MSM identity brings with it a set of unique stigmas based on the combination of those identities. Furthermore, the stigmatization of homosexuality may be enhanced if Black MSM have low social class or HIV (Nelson, Walker, DuBois, & Giwa, 2013). Black MSM who are HIV-positive experience additional stigma based on their status, including hindrance of open sexual communication and less closeness with the gay community (Bird & Voisin, 2013). Although the manifestations may vary, many Black MSM attribute the intra-racial stigma they experience to the influence of negative rhetoric in many Black religious spaces that is propagated by religious doctrine, family members, and peers (Miller, 2007; Wilson et al., 2015).

In keeping with the tenets of intersectionality, it is important to note that some identities can be advantageous while others are simultaneously seen as a disadvantage (Bowleg, 2012; Wilson et al., 2015). The male identity concerning Black MSM has its privileges while being Black and gay are perceived as strikes based on societal norms (Bowleg 2012). Additionally, the identities that make up Black MSM are not static; new identities may emerge while others may become more prominent due to changing social and environmental circumstances. For example, a Black MSM who relocates from the rural U.S. South to the urban Northeast may experience a shift in regional identity in order to assimilate into their new environment, or maintain a strong identification with his regional identity of origin. The intersectional experience of Black MSM warrants further attention because Black MSM possess privileged and stigmatized identities in one body and not all of these identities are addressed within existing HIV prevention and care initiatives (Bowleg, 2012; Wilson et al., 2015).

Empirical Applications of Intersectionality with Black MSM

Here we provide two examples of studies that used intersectional approaches to better understand factors related to HIV infection among Black MSM in specific geographic contexts. The first study (*Sexual Health in Faith Traditions [SHIFT] Study*) is a quantitative study examining psychosocial factors associated with sexual behaviors among Black MSM in the Deep South[2] (Smallwood, Spencer, Ingram, Thrasher, & Thompson-Robinson, 2015, 2016). In particular, this study examined how certain psychosocial factors may manifest differently for Black MSM than they do for other racial/ethnic groups of MSM, and how these factors then influence engagement in safer sex behaviors. The second study (*Giving Voice to Black Gay & Bisexual Men in the South: A Qualitative Inquiry*) was a qualitative investigation of factors influencing mental and sexual health outcomes among Black MSM in central South Carolina. In this study, intersectional analysis was used to understand differences in Black MSM experiences based on certain characteristics, showing the diversity of experiences among members of this group. Although neither of these studies focused specifically on rural Black MSM, the findings of each can be used to inform future research and practice in rural settings.

Sexual Health in Faith Traditions (SHIFT) Study

The purpose of the SHIFT Study was to examine the ways in which religiosity, spirituality, and internalized homonegativity (IH) are associated with engagement in sexual risk behaviors among Black MSM living in the Deep South region of the U.S. The study was conceptualized in response to a dearth of intersectional approaches used to explore factors related to HIV risk among Black MSM in the Deep South, where HIV rates remain extremely high. For example, although IH had been identified as a risk factor for HIV infection, few studies had examined how IH manifested in the lives of Black MSM in the South, or the factors that contributed to the development of IH among Black MSM. Similarly, little research had examined the impact of social structural factors, such as the "Black church," on the sexual

---

[2]The "Deep South" region was defined as the states of Alabama, Georgia, Louisiana, Mississippi, North Carolina, and South Carolina.

behaviors of Black MSM. To that end, the SHIFT Study sought to address the relative invisibility of the lived experiences of southern Black MSM and Black social structures from our HIV prevention discourse.

The SHIFT Study was a cross-sectional quantitative study of Black MSM living in the Deep South. Black men living in the Deep South, ages 18 years and older who self-reported being gay, bisexual, or having sex with a man in the previous 12 months were eligible to participate for a total sample of 348 Black MSM in the study. Details regarding the study's methods can be found in other sources (Smallwood et al., 2015, 2016).

The first research aim examined the structure of IH among Black MSM. Using the 23-item Internalized Homonegativity Inventory (IHNI; Mayfield, 2001), participants were asked to respond to a series of statements measuring IH across three dimensions: Personal Homonegativity, or negative emotions and attitudes toward one's own sexuality; Gay Affirmation, or the degree to which one's same-sex orientation is viewed as positive and fulfilling; and Morality of Homosexuality, or "negative attitudes regarding the moral implications of same-sex behavior and attraction" (Mayfield, 2001, p. 67). These dimensions were based on initial research conducted with predominantly White MSM living in the Midwest; however, exploratory factor analysis revealed a different dimensional structure of IH among Black MSM. While the Gay Affirmation component stayed intact, the Personal Homonegativity and Morality of Homosexuality dimensions merged to form one component. This finding suggests that, for Black MSM in the South, it is difficult for them to separate their personal negative feelings about their sexuality from negative social stereotypes about homosexuality. This finding has significant implications for HIV prevention interventions focusing on Black MSM. If an intervention plans to address IH as a risk factor, then the discussion of IH may not just focus on personal feelings, but it may also address broader negative stereotypes and misconceptions about homosexuality that exist in the communities where Black MSM live, work, pray, and play.

The second research aim examined the overall relationships between religiosity, spirituality, IH, and condom use among Black MSM. Almost half of respondents reported using condoms every time they engaged in anal sex as the insertive or receptive partner. The study found that greater religious commitment was associated with higher IH scores, while greater personal spirituality was associated with lower IH scores. Surprisingly, higher IH was associated with more frequent condom use. There are many potential factors that might influence this relationship. For one, Black MSM already experience stigma and discrimination based on their racial and sexual identities; therefore, Black MSM with higher levels of IH may use condoms more frequently not only to avoid becoming infected with HIV, but also the additional level of stigma that would accompany such a diagnosis.

The results of this study illustrate the importance of using an intersectional lens to examine factors related to HIV risk among Black MSM. For example, the finding that IH manifests differently for Black MSM than for other racial and ethnic MSM is indicative of how Black MSM's sexual identity is influenced by their racial identity. Therefore, the use of "one size fits all" approaches to address HIV-related risk and protective factors among MSM in general may not be effective for Black MSM because their existence at that intersection changes the way in which those factors are experienced. Furthermore, the findings from the second research study aim to demonstrate the ways in which multiple stigmas can affect the psychological, social, and behavioral outcomes of Black MSM. Based on these findings, incorporating experiences with stigma and discrimination into HIV prevention initiatives for Black MSM could prove beneficial. By centering the lived experiences of Black MSM into future HIV prevention research and intervention development, we can gain a clearer understanding of the most salient factors associated with HIV risk and protection for this population.

Giving Voice to Black Gay and Bisexual Men in the South: A Qualitative Inquiry

As evidence builds behind the use of intersectional frameworks, some public health researchers are incorporating the framework into studies examining the impact of HIV-related health outcomes among Black MSM. One study conducted among a sample of self-identifying Black gay and bisexual men ($n = 32$) in Columbia, South Carolina explored the influences of religion, spirituality, and family dynamics on the mental health and sexual behaviors of Black MSM (Carter, 2014). The aims of the study were to identify sources of psychological distress that Black MSM experienced that place them at risk for engaging in condomless anal intercourse (CAI) based upon the literature demonstrating a positive association between psychological distress and CAI (Crawford, Allison, Zamboni, & Soto, 2002; Ibañez, Purcell, Stall, Parsons, & Gómez, 2005; Myers, Javanbakht, Martinez, & Obediah, 2003; Parsons, Halkitis, Wolitski, Gómez, & Study Team, 2003; Stokes and Peterson 1998). This study is one of few qualitative inquiries examining and describing the contextual experiences of Black MSM in the South and HIV-related outcomes. Findings from the Carter study indicated that family and religion were a major source of distress for the sample of men independently and collectively. Depending upon the man's upbringing, social support, and resiliency, encounters with family and/or religion due to disapproval of their sexuality or non-conforming gender roles exacerbated the psychological distress experienced. In some situations, men who exhibited drastic encounters with racial and sexuality discrimination were more apt to engage in risky sexual behaviors like CAI in comparison to other men in the study.

The Carter study highlights the importance of unpacking system-level barriers (e.g., social and institutional racism) that many minority communities face when trying to protect themselves from HIV or receive quality care for HIV treatment. Using an intersectional framework not only provided an in-depth understanding of the social and contextual factors influencing the lived experiences of the men in the study, but it also aided with developing interview questions and data analysis processes. For instance, the interview guide contained questions that were specific to learning more about the identities of being a Black gay or bisexual man collectively and individually. Some examples of the questions include the following: (1) *How do you think being Black has caused you stress in your life? Being a man? Being gay (or whatever word you choose to use);* (2) *how do you think being Black has benefited you in your life? Being a man? Being gay (or whatever word you choose to use)?; and* (3) *which is most important to you: being Black, being a man, being gay (or whatever word you choose to use)? Why?* Although some questions were focused on single identity of the respondents, many of the respondents were unable to disassociate one identity from another, which was important during the data analysis portion of this study. The intersectional framework assisted with understanding the dynamic interactions of their multiple identities and provided additional context to how those identities manifest in their lives and impacted their mental and sexual health outcomes. Data collection and analysis of this study was the impetus for the generation of additional questions regarding how to apply intersectional frameworks in practical settings particularly among providers serving Black MSM. For example, many study participants reflected on experiences of discrimination when interacting with HIV prevention service providers due to their sexual orientation. The experiences of these men provided insight on the need for culturally sensitive and appropriate interventions targeting providers who service or care for Black MSM and the need for additional research that incorporates an intersectional framework in the research design and analytical approaches among this population.

Intersectionality—The Way Forward

Now that we have provided an overview of intersectionality and empirical evidence demonstrating the application of intersectionality in research studies among Black MSM, we offer discussion on future directions of utilizing this framework in research and practice specifically for those in rural settings. Given the high degree of diversity within Black MSM communities and the disproportionate HIV rates among them in the South, there are multiple opportunities to employ intersectional approaches with this population at multiple levels.

First, we acknowledge that the studies discussed in this chapter took place in a more general Southern context, and may not be specific to the experiences of rural-dwelling Black MSM. However, there is significant overlap between characteristics of rural communities and the overall culture of the South. For example, the primacy of religious values and experience is a characteristic that has been noted in Southern communities and in rural communities nationwide (Dillon & Savage, 2006). The inclusion of these studies is not meant to be an exhaustive description of the experiences of rural-dwelling Black MSM; however, these studies do provide a starting point for understanding the complex interplay of social, cultural, and historical factors that contribute to HIV risk for Black MSM.

We understand that intersectionality can be a difficult concept to fully grasp, let alone incorporate into HIV prevention practice; however, there are multiple ways in which an intersectional lens can be infused into HIV prevention and care work. For example, cultural competence training can serve as an entry point into intersectional practice. Black MSM often have had negative experiences with racial discrimination, homophobia, heterosexism, and HIV-related stigma within and outside of healthcare settings (Bogart, Landrine, Galvin, & Wagner, 2013; Irvin et al., 2014). To overcome barriers related to these experiences, the public health workforce should be culturally competent and create environments that are culturally appropriate and sensitive to the needs of this diverse population. For example, it is very easy to instruct a Black MSM to take medication to treat or prevent HIV, but if he has experienced a stigmatizing or discriminatory incident with his healthcare provider or the healthcare setting based on his race, sexuality, or both, he may be less likely to engage in HIV prevention or care initiatives specific to his needs, thus exposing a major structural barrier. It is important to be conscious of both the physical and social environment of healthcare spaces, and make sure they are as devoid of stigmatizing images, messages, and dialogue as possible. Cultural competence training is a useful tool to aid in this practice. Also, while it is essential for primary care physicians and other primary healthcare providers to exhibit cultural appropriateness, ancillary staff who have direct contact with Black MSM clients are also a vital component of the healthcare experience. Therefore, frontline staff such as receptionists, medical assistants, etc. should also exhibit a high level of cultural appropriateness when serving this population.

In addition to general cultural competence in practice, using an intersectional framework in a practical setting can assist providers with identifying, recognizing, and ultimately modifying any biases they may have about a particular group of people. This can be accomplished through staff assessments, trainings, and professional development opportunities that seek to identify personal biases toward certain groups, understand why they exist, and develop solutions to reduce them in order to improve the standard of care given to marginalized communities like Black MSM.

Community-based participatory approaches can also be used to better understand the lived experiences of Black MSM. Interviews, focus groups, and forums with Black MSM in a rural service area can be a helpful way to identify issues and factors specific to that local context. The information gained from local inquiry can then be infused into existing HIV prevention interventions, and linkage to and retention in HIV care to improve effectiveness. These approaches are also strategies to affirm the lived experiences of Black MSM in that local area and to engage and empower them as local collaborative partners in HIV prevention and care efforts.

Just as there is diversity among Black MSM and these men have distinctive lived experiences, the same respect should be extended to transgender populations. While transgender individuals were not the priority population of discussion for this chapter, they have their own set of unique experiences and needs that require similar attention as Black MSM and should not be lumped into a category with any type of MSM (Melendez, Bonem, & Sember, 2006; Keller, 2009). While there is limited research and examples of engaging transgender populations, utilization of intersectional frameworks can provide an opportunity to learn and empower this community as well.

Intersectionality is not the "cure" for ending racism, poverty, heterosexism, and other social ills that exacerbate health outcomes in general; however, it does offer a mechanism for examining existing forces that can adversely affect health-related outcomes. In the context of HIV, this framework can yield more expansive understanding of site-specific or geographically specific issues that hinder Black MSM from obtaining the quality services and care that they deserve. Furthermore, applying an intersectional lens to HIV prevention work creates additional opportunities to develop interventions that will assist us in achieving the third NHAS goal of reducing HIV-related disparities. Many of the experiences shared about Black MSM touch on problems related to racism, homophobia, stigma, educational and employment opportunities, and unfair distribution of resources. As we charge our way forward, HIV prevention efforts should be better equipped to address the collective issues Black MSM encounter daily in hopes of reducing the HIV disparity within this population. If intersectionality does anything, it demonstrates how complex we are as human beings and while there may not be a "one-size fits all model," this framework generates a space to become more creative in our approaches to HIV prevention among many of the marginalized communities in this country and generates a vessel for recognizing and appreciating their truth.

Disclaimer

The findings and conclusions in this report are those of the author and do not necessarily represent the official position of the Centers for Disease Control and Prevention.

References

Association for Women's Rights in Development. (2004). Intersectionality: A tool for gender and economic justice. *Women's Rights and Economic Change, 9,* 1–8.

Badgett, M. V., Durso, L. E., & Schneebaum, A. (2013). *New patterns of poverty in the lesbian, gay, and bisexual community.* Los Angeles, CA: Williams Institute, University of California-Los Angeles. Accessed from http://williamsinstitute.law.ucla.edu/wp-content/uploads/LGB-Poverty-Update-Jun-2013.pdf

Bauer, G. R. (2014). Incorporating intersectionality theory into population health research methodology: Challenges and the potential to advance health equity. *Social Science and Medicine, 110,* 10–17.

Beatty, L. A., Wheeler, D., & Gaiter, J. (2004). HIV prevention research for African Americans: Current and future directions. *The Journal of Black Psychology, 30,* 40–58.

Bird, J. D., & Voisin, D. R. (2013). "You're an open target to be abused": A qualitative study of stigma and HIV self-disclosure among Black men who have sex with men. *American Journal of Public Health, 103,* 2193–2199.

Bogart, L. M., Landrine, H., Galvan, F. H., Wagner, G. J., & Klein, D. J. (2013). Perceived discrimination and physical health among HIV-positive Black and Latino men who have sex with men. *AIDS and Behavior, 17*(4), 1431–1441.

Bowleg, L. (2012). The problem with the phrase women and minorities: intersectionality—an important theoretical framework for public health. *American Journal of Public Health, 102*(7), 1267–1273.

Bowleg, L. (2013). "Once you've blended the cake, you can't take the parts back to the main ingredients": Black gay and bisexual men's descriptions and experiences of intersectionality. *Sex Roles, 68*(11–12), 754–767.

Bowleg, L., Teti, M., Malebranche, D. J., & Tschann, J. M. (2013). "It's an uphill battle everyday": Intersectionality, low-income Black heterosexual men, and implications for HIV prevention research and interventions. *Psychology of Men and Masculinity, 14,* 25–34.

Carter, J.W, & Simmons, D.S. (2014). Two strikes and you're out!: The implications of race, gender, and sexuality on the mental health and sexual behaviors of Black gay and bisexual men. *Paper presented at the meeting of the American Anthropological Association,* Washington, D.C.

CDC. (2011). *High-impact prevention: CDC's approach to reducing HIV infections in the United States.* Retrieved from http://www.cdc.gov/hiv/strategy/dhap/pdf/nhas_booklet.pdf

CDC. (2014a). *Pre-exposure prophylaxis (PrEP) for HIV prevention.* Retrieved from http://www.cdc.gov/hiv/pdf/prep_fact_sheet_final.pdf

CDC. (2014b). *Pre-exposure prophylaxis for the prevention of HIV infection in the United States-2014: A clinical practice guideline.* Atlanta, GA: Centers for Disease Control and Prevention.

CDC. (2015a). *HIV in the United States: At a glance.* Retrieved from http://www.cdc.gov/hiv/pdf/statistics/overview/hiv-at-a-glance-factsheet.pdf

CDC. (2015b). HIV surveillance report: Diagnoses of HIV infection in the United States and dependent areas, 2014 (Vol. 26, pp. 1–123). Atlanta, GA: Centers for Disease Control and Prevention.

CDC. (2016a). *HIV in the Southern United States.* Retrieved from https://www.cdc.gov/hiv/pdf/policies/cdc-hiv-in-the-south-issue-brief.pdf

CDC. (2016b). Prevention benefits of HIV treatment. Retrieved from http://www.cdc.gov/hiv/research/biomedicalresearch/tap/index.html

Cochran, S. D., Sullivan, J. G., & Mays, V. M. (2003). Prevalence of mental disorders, psychological distress, and mental health services use among lesbian, gay, and bisexual adults in the United States. *Journal of Consulting and Clinical Psychology, 71*(1), 53.

Cole, E. R. (2009). Intersectionality and research in psychology. *The American Psychologist, 64*(3), 170–180.

Crawford, I., Allison, K. W., Zamboni, B. D., & Soto, T. (2002). The influence of dual-identity development on the psychosocial functioning of African-American gay and bisexual men. *Journal of Sex Research, 39*(3), 179–189.

Crenshaw, K. (1989). Demarginalizing the intersection of race and sex: A black feminist critique of antidiscrimination doctrine, feminist theory and antiracist politics. *U. Chi. Legal F.,* 139.

Crenshaw, K. (1991). Mapping the margins: Intersectionality, identity politics, and violence against women of color. *Stanford law review,* 1241–1299.

Dentato, M. P. (2012). *The minority stress perspective. Psychology & AIDS Exchange* (Vol. 37, pp. 12–15). Washington, D.C.: American Psychological Association (Spring Issue).

Dillon, M., & Savage, S. (2006). Values and religion in rural America: Attitudes toward abortion and same-sex relations. *The Carsey School of Public Policy at the Scholars' Repository.* Paper 12. Accessed from http://scholars.unh.edu/carsey/12

DiPlacido, J. (1998). *Minority stress among lesbians, gay men, and bisexuals: A consequence of heterosexism, homophobia, and stigmatization.* Sage Publications, Inc.

Dottolo, A. L., & Stewart, A. J. (2008). "Don't ever forget now, you're a Black man in America": Intersections of race, class and gender in encounters with the police. *Sex Roles, 59*(5–6), 350–364.

Dowshen, N., Binns, H. J., & Garofalo, R. (2009). Experiences of HIV-related stigma among young men who have sex with men. *AIDS Patient Care & STDs, 23*(5), 371–376.

Fisher, J. D., & Smith, L. (2009). Secondary prevention of HIV infection: The current state of prevention for positives. *Current Opinion in HIV and AIDS, 4*(4), 279–287.

Friedman, E. M., Williams, D. R., Singer, B. H., & Ryff, C. D. (2009). Chronic discrimination predicts higher circulating levels of E-selectin in a national sample: The MIDUS study. *Brain, Behavior, and Immunity, 23*(5), 684–692.

Fullilove, M. M., Fullilove, E. R., West, C., Wilson, P., & Wright, J. J. (1997). *Though I stand at the door and knock: Discussions on the Black church struggle with homosexuality & AIDS*. Paper presented at the Though I Stand at the Door and Knock, New York City.

Glick, S. N., & Golden, M. R. (2010). Persistence of racial differences in attitudes toward homosexuality in the United States. *Jaids-Journal of Acquired Immune Deficiency Syndromes, 55*(4), 516–523.

Grant, R. M., Lama, J. R., Anderson, P. L., McMahan, V., Liu, A. Y., Vargas, L., … Glidden, D. V. (2010). Preexposure chemoprophylaxis for HIV prevention in men who have sex with men. *New England Journal of Medicine, 363*(27), 2587–2599. doi:10.1056/NEJMoa1011205

Haile, R., Padilla, M. B., & Parker, E. A. (2011). "Stuck in the quagmire of an HIV ghetto": The meaning of stigma in the lives of older Black gay and bisexual men living with HIV in New York City. *Culture, Health, and Sexuality, 13*, 429–442.

Harawa, N. T., & Ford, C. L. (2009). The foundation of modern racial categories and implications for research on black/white disparities in health. *Ethnicity and Disease, 19*(2), 209–217.

Harding, S. G. (2004). *The feminist standpoint theory reader: Intellectual and political controversies*. Psychology Press.

Hatzenbuehler, M. L. (2009). How does sexual minority stigma "get under the skin"? A psychological mediation framework. *Psychological Bulletin, 135*(5), 707.

Ibañez, G. E., Purcell, D. W., Stall, R., Parsons, J. T., & Gómez, C. A. (2005). Sexual risk, substance use, and psychological distress in HIV-positive gay and bisexual men who also inject drugs. *AIDS, 19*, S49–S55.

Irvin, R., Wilton, L., Scott, H., Beauchamp, G., Wang, L., Betancourt, J., … Buchbinder, S. (2014). A study of perceived racial discrimination in Black men who have sex with men (MSM) and its association with healthcare utilization and HIV testing. *AIDS and Behavior, 18*(7), 1272–1278.

Jones, C. P. (2000). Levels of racism: A theoretic framework and a gardener's tale. *American Journal of Public Health, 90*(8), 1212–1215.

Jones, K. T., Wilton, L., Millett, G. A., & Johnson, W. D. (2010). Formulating the stress and severity model of minority social stress for Black men who have sex with men. In D. H. McCree, K. T. Jones, & A. O'Leary (Eds.), *African Americans and HIV/AIDS: Understanding and addressing the epidemic* (pp. 223–238). New York: Springer.

Kennedy, C., & Fonner, V. (2014). Pre-exposure prophylaxis for men who have sex with men: a systematic review. In *Consolidated guidelines on HIV prevention, diagnosis, treatment and care for key populations*. Geneva: World Health Organization; Annex 1.

Keller, K. (2009). Transgender health and HIV. *BETA: Bulletin of Experimental Treatments for AIDS: A Publication of the San Francisco AIDS Foundation, 21*(4), 40–50.

Krieger, N., Chen, J. T., Waterman, P. D., Hartman, C., Stoddard, A. M., Quinn, M. M., … Barbeau, E. M. (2008). The inverse hazard law: Blood pressure, sexual harassment, racial discrimination, workplace abuse and occupational exposures in US low-income black, white and Latino workers. *Social Science & Medicine, 67*(12), 1970–1981.

Lemelle, A. J., & Battle, J. (2004). Black masculinity matters in attitudes toward gay males. *Journal of Homosexuality, 47*(1), 39–51.

Lewis, G. B. (2003). Black-White differences in attitudes toward homosexuality and gay rights. *The Public Opinion Quarterly, 67*(1), 59–78.

Mayfield, W. (2001). The development of an internalized homonegativity inventory for gay men. *Journal of Homosexuality, 41*(2), 53–76.

Mays, V. M., & Cochran, S. D. (2001). Mental health correlates of perceived discrimination among lesbian, gay, and bisexual adults in the United States. *American Journal of Public Health, 91*(11), 1869–1876.

Mays, V. M., Cochran, S. D., & Zamudio, A. (2004). HIV prevention research: Are we meeting the needs of African-American men who have sex with men? *Journal of Black Psychology,* 78–105.

Melendez, R., Bonem, L., & Sember, R. (2006). On bodies and research: Transgender issues in health and HIV research articles. *Sexuality Research & Social Policy, 3*(4), 21–38.

Meyer, I. H. (1995). Minority stress and mental health in gay men. *Journal of health and social behavior,* 38–56.

Meyer, I. H. (2003). Prejudice, social stress, and mental health in lesbian, gay, and bisexual populations: Conceptual issues and research evidence. *Psychological Bulletin, 129*(5), 674.

Miller, M., Serner, M., & Wagner, M. (2005). Sexual diversity among Black men who have sex with men in an inner-city community. *Journal of Urban Health: Bulletin of the New York Academy of Medicine, 82,* 26–34.

Miller, R. L. (2007). Legacy denied: African American gay men, AIDS, and the Black church. *Social Work, 52,* 51–61.

Millett, G. A., Flores, S. A., Peterson, J. L., & Bakeman, R. (2007a). Explaining disparities in HIV infection among black and white men who have sex with men: A meta-analysis of HIV risk behaviors. *AIDS, 21*(15), 2083–2091.

Millett, G. A., Malebranche, D., & Peterson, J. L. (2007b). HIV/AIDS prevention research among Black men who have sex with men: Current progress and future directions. In I. H. Meyer & M. E. Northridge (Eds.), *The health of sexual minorities: Public health perspectives on lesbian, gay, bisexual and transgender populations* (pp. 539–565). Boston, MA: Springer, US.

Millett, G. A., Peterson, J. L., Flores, S. A., Hart, T. A., Jeffries, W. L., 4th, Wilson, P. A., et al. (2012). Comparisons of disparities and risks of HIV infection in black and other men who have sex with men in Canada, UK, and USA: A meta-analysis. *The Lancet, 380*(9839), 341–348.

Myers, H. F., Javanbakht, M., Martinez, M., & Obediah, S. (2003). Psychosocial predictors of risky sexual behaviors in African American men: Implications for prevention. *AIDS Education and Prevention, 15,* 66.

National HIV/AIDS Strategy for the United States. (2010). Retrieved from http://www.whitehouse.gov/sites/default/files/uploads/NHAS.pdf

National Institute on Drug Abuse. (2012). What is HAART? Retrieved from https://www.drugabuse.gov/publications/research-reports/hivaids/what-haart

Nelson, L. E., Walker, J. J., DuBois, S. N., & Giwa, S. (2013). Your blues ain't like mine: Considering integrative antiracism in HIV prevention research with Black men who have sex with men in Canada and the United States. *Nursing Inquiry, 21*(4), 270–282.

Parker, R., & Aggleton, P. (2003). HIV and AIDS-related stigma and discrimination: A conceptual framework and implications for action. *Social Science and Medicine, 57,* 13–24.

Parsons, J. T., Halkitis, P. N., Wolitski, R. J., Gómez, C. A., & Study Team, T. S. U. M. s. (2003). Correlates of sexual risk behaviors among HIV-positive men who have sex with men. *AIDS Education and Prevention, 15*(5), 383–400.

Peterson, J. L., & Jones, K. T. (2009). HIV prevention for Black men who have sex with men in the United States. *American Journal of Public Health, 99*(6), 976–980.

Rasmussen, A. C. (2014). Toward an intersectional political science pedagogy. *Journal of Political Science Education, 10*(1), 102–116.

Reif, S., Pence, B., Hall, I., Hu, X., Whetten, K., & Wilson, E. (2015). HIV diagnoses, prevalence and outcomes in nine southern states. *Journal of Community Health, 40*(4), 642–651.

Reif, S., Whetten, K., Wilson, E. R., McAllaster, C., Pence, B. W., Legrand, S., & Gong, W. (2014). HIV/AIDS in the Southern USA: A disproportionate epidemic. *AIDS Care, 26*(3), 351–359. doi:10.1080/09540121.2013.824535

Smallwood, S. W., Spencer, S. M., Annang Ingram, L., Thrasher, J. F., & Thompson-Robinson, M. (2016). Different dimensions: Internalized homonegativity among African American men who have sex with men. *Journal of Homosexuality, 64*(1), 45–60. doi:10.1080/00918369.2016. 1172869

Smallwood, S. W., Spencer, S. M., Annang Ingram, L., Thrasher, J. F., & Thompson-Robinson, M. (2015). Examining the relationships between religiosity, spirituality, internalized homonegativity, and condom use among African American men who have sex with men. *American Journal of Men's Health*. [epub ahead of print]. doi:10.1177/1557988315590835

Stokes, J. P., & Peterson, J. L. (1998). Homophobia, self-esteem, and risk for HIV among African American men who have sex with men. *AIDS Education and Prevention, 10*(3), 278–292.

Tobin, K. E., Cutchin, M., Latkin, C. A., & Takahashi, L. M. (2013). Social geographies of African American men who have sex with men (MSM): A qualitative exploration of the social, spatial, and temporal context of HIV risk in Baltimore, Maryland. *Health and Place, 22,* 1–6.

Vincent, W., Peterson, J., & Parrott, D. (2009). Differences in African American and White women's attitudes toward lesbians and gay men. *Sex Roles, 61*(9), 599–606.

Weber, L. (2010). *Understanding race, class, gender, and sexuality: A conceptual framework.* New York: Oxford University Press Inc.

Williams, D. R., & Mohammed, S. A. (2009). Discrimination and racial disparities in health: Evidence and needed research. *Journal of Behavioral Medicine, 32*(1), 20–47.

Wilson, P. A., Valera, P., Martos, A. J., Wittlin, N. M., Muñoz-Laboy, & Parker, R. G. (2015). Contributions of qualitative research in informing HIV/AIDS interventions targeting Black MSM in the United States. *Journal of Sex Research, 0*(0), 1–13.

Chapter 10
Learning to Age Successfully with HIV

Barbara J. Blake and Gloria Ann Jones Taylor

When the HIV epidemic began more than 30 years ago, people diagnosed with AIDS were only expected to live 1–2 years. However, the introduction of effective antiretroviral (ARV) treatment in the 1990s transitioned HIV disease from a death sentence to a chronic illness. Today, individuals who are diagnosed early, receive ARVs, and maintain a suppressed viral load can conceivably have a life expectancy similar to their HIV-negative counterparts (Samji et al., 2013). Because of the success in treating HIV, it is currently estimated that one-fourth of the 1.2 million people living with the disease in the United States are 55 years of age and older (Centers for Disease Control and Prevention [CDC], 2016).

Despite effective treatment for HIV disease, age-related chronic illnesses are more common among individuals living with long-standing infection. The majority of these physical health conditions include cardiovascular disease, osteoporosis, non-AIDS defining cancers, and diabetes (Cardoso et al., 2013). In addition to physical health problems, aging with HIV increases vulnerability to mental health complications, such as depression and impaired neurocognitive functioning (Rueda, Law, & Rourke, 2014).

Aging is a biological fact: the body will decline mentally and physically over time and the aging process varies from person to person. Adopting and maintaining a healthy lifestyle that extends into later years can contribute to people aging successfully. The purpose of this chapter is to review key theories related to successful aging and HIV, discuss physical and mental health conditions that are common among people aging with HIV, and offer recommendations for how healthcare providers can help people age successfully with the disease.

B.J. Blake (✉) · G.A.J. Taylor
WellStar School of Nursing, Kennesaw State University,
520 Parliament Garden Way, Kennesaw, GA 30144, USA
e-mail: bblake@kennesaw.edu

G.A.J. Taylor
e-mail: gtaylor@kennesaw.edu

© Springer International Publishing AG 2017
F.M. Parks et al. (eds.), *HIV/AIDS in Rural Communities*,
DOI 10.1007/978-3-319-56239-1_10

Theories of Successful Aging

Rowe and Kahan's (1998) theoretical conception of aging is three-dimensional: avoidance or low risk of disease, maintenance of cognitive and physical capacity, and active social engagement. The primary premise is to age successfully by maintaining both mental and physical functionings into old age. Their theoretical perspective generated a great deal of research and popularized the notion of successful aging (Martin et al., 2015). However, many find this theory to be problematic, as this model excludes disability or loss of function. Also, there is limited consideration for social and environmental factors. More importantly, factors related to the spiritual realm are not addressed (Topaz, Troutman-Jordan, & MacKenzie, 2014).

Another model that addresses successful aging was developed by Baltes and Baltes (1990). This model examines the development of adults as they progress through life. To age successfully, the model proposes that a person will decide on goals based on available internal and external resources within their environment; engage in behaviors that will enhance available resources; and consciously select behaviors and goals that allow for adequate functioning (Donnellan & O'Neill, 2014).

As people age, they may face physical, social, and environmental challenges. Kahana and Kahana's (1996) stress-theory-based framework of preventive and corrective proactivity supports this perspective on aging. This model allows for facing the stressors of normative age-related stressors of chronic illness, social losses, and lack of person–environment fit. Successful aging is possible as individuals utilize internal coping resources and external social resources to enhance quality of life through proactive behavioral adaptation (Martin et al., 2015). In this model, proactive behavioral adaptation can embrace numerous activities; for example, health promotion, seeking support, planning ahead, reaching out to others, and modification of the environment. This model has been applied to vulnerable populations, such as persons living and aging with HIV. According to Kahana and Kahana (2001), their "conceptualization stresses social and psychological states and indicators of a high quality of life … and also emphasizes finding meaning in life, as an important quality of life outcome …" (p. S54).

While the discussion above does not address all theoretical conceptualizations of successful aging, it is clear that informative models exist and all suggest attributes that can be used to guide positive health interventions to support older persons living with chronic diseases, including persons living with HIV. Successful aging means maintaining good health both physical and mental, which entails engaging in physical activity, eating well, seeing a doctor as recommended, keeping connected with friends and family, and meeting personal spiritual/faith needs.

Physical Health and Aging with HIV

Cardiovascular Disease

People living with HIV are 1.5–2 times more likely to develop cardiovascular disease (CVD) compared to the general population. The explanation for this increased risk encompasses a complex interplay between biology and environment. Biological risk factors include the length of time someone is infected, elevated cholesterol and/or triglycerides (dyslipidemia) related to antiretroviral therapy (particularly protease inhibitors), abdominal fat accumulation, and altered glucose metabolism. Recent evidence has identified that persistent immune activation and chronic inflammation associated with HIV infection are also major contributors to CVD, because both lead to the accumulation of atypical plaque in the cardiovascular system (Triant, 2013). More traditional biological and environmental risk factors for CVD such as smoking, lack of exercise, lifestyle, obesity, and genetics also compound the problem. Recommendations for treating dyslipidemia among people living with HIV include lifestyle changes such as increased exercise and diet modification. In addition, persons who are taking ARVs that increase cholesterol and/or triglyceride levels should discuss making a HIV medication change with their healthcare provider. If these modifications are not effective, cholesterol and/or triglyceride lowering medication that is safe can be considered (Monroe et al., 2015).

As within the general population, hypertension is a significant contributor to CVD among people aging with HIV. Factors associated with the development of hypertension in people living with HIV are similar to those found in HIV-negative people: older age, family history, excess body weight, physical inactivity, excessive alcohol consumption, tobacco use, and unhealthy eating habits. HIV-specific factors such as disease severity, length of time living with the disease, and disease treatment on the development of hypertension have been reported, but findings are not conclusive. The goals for managing hypertension in the aging HIV population are similar to those in the general population; however, prescribing providers should be aware of potential drug interactions (Manner, Baekken, Oektedalen, & Os, 2012).

It is important that healthcare providers ascertain an individual's risk for CVD and offer recommendations and/or treatment as necessary. The Framingham Risk Score (FRS) and Prospective Cardiovascular Münster (PROCAM) score are often used to estimate risk of CVD within the general population. However, the use of these instruments to accurately measure CVD risk among people living with HIV has been debated (Costa & Almeida, 2015; Nery et al., 2013).

Family history (genetic background) along with lifestyle (diet and exercise) are measures used to assess the risk of developing CVD. Individuals cannot change genetic predisposition, but can modify their lifestyle. Healthcare providers need to educate all adults about nutritious eating, maintaining a healthy weight, getting regular exercise, limiting alcohol, and not smoking. Changes in these areas of a person's life can help prevent or control many chronic diseases.

Osteoporosis

Among older adults living with HIV, osteoporosis (thinning of the bone) has been found to occur at a rate that is more than 3 times greater than the rate within the general population. Women are more likely to develop osteoporosis after menopause because estrogen, a hormone that protects against bone loss, decreases sharply. In addition to risk factors shared with the general population for osteoporosis (low body mass, sedentary lifestyle, smoking, alcohol use, and decreased intake of calcium and vitamin D), other risk factors for loss of bone mass directly related to HIV include immune disregulation, chronic inflammation, and initiation of ARV treatment (Short, Shaw, Fisher, Walker-Bone, & Gilleece, 2014).

For people living with HIV it is recommended that men 50 years of age or older, postmenopausal women, individuals with a history of fracture or receiving glucocorticoid treatment, and persons with one or more risk factors for fracture, be screened for loss of bone mineral density using dual X-ray absorptiometry (DXA) of the spine and hip. To reduce or prevent the incidence of osteoporosis, calcium and vitamin D supplements, smoking cessation, decreased alcohol usage, and weight-bearing exercises should be recommended. Prescription medications that slow or prevent bone loss are also available (Mallon, 2014).

Non-AIDS Defining Cancers

AIDS defining cancers such as non-Hodgkin lymphoma, cervical cancer, and Kaposi sarcoma are declining, while non-AIDS defining cancers, such as anal and lung cancer, are on the rise (Silverberg et al., 2015). People infected with HIV are 25 times more likely to be diagnosed with anal cancer than uninfected people, 5 times as likely to be diagnosed with liver cancer, 3 times as likely to be diagnosed with lung cancer, and approximately 10 times more likely to be diagnosed with Hodgkin lymphoma (Grulich, van Leeuwen, Falster, & Vajdic, 2007). This increased incidence is because of an aging HIV population and a weakened immune system that reduces the body's ability to fight agents that might lead to cancer. Patients infected with HIV often present with an earlier onset and have worse outcomes than non-HIV-infected patients with the same cancer diagnosis (National Cancer Institute [NCI], 2011).

Anal cancer is caused by human papillomavirus (HPV), a sexually transmitted infection that resides in the outermost layer of the skin or mucous membranes. This virus is the most prevalent sexually transmitted infection in the United States. Men who have anal sex with men (MSM) are more likely to get anal HPV than men who only have sex with women. The prevalence of anal HPV among men who only have sex with women is around 15% while anal HPV prevalence for MSM is about 60% (NCI, 2015; Sadlier et al., 2014).

At this time, there are no national recommendations for routine anal cancer screening. Some HIV specialists recommend that anal cytologic screening (anal Pap) be offered to HIV-positive men and women. However, anal Paps should not be done without the availability of referral for high-resolution anoscopy. An anoscopy uses an instrument for closer examination and evaluation of the anus and rectum (Department of Health and Human Services, 2016). Because there is limited data about the benefits of anal Pap screening, randomized controlled studies are needed to determine if Pap screening will reduce the morbidity and mortality of anal cancer among people living with HIV.

Approximately, 19% of adults in the United States are smokers. However, the rate of smoking among adults who are HIV positive is 2–3 times higher than the general population. Among people living with HIV, the average age of diagnosis with lung cancer is mid to late forties and most people are symptomatic when diagnosed. Studies have found that even after adjusting for factors such as smoking duration and intensity, lung cancer is 2–4 times greater among HIV-infected persons as compared to the general population (Palacios et al., 2014). Health education, smoking cessation, and early detection are critical as lung cancer can be more aggressive in adults living with HIV.

People aging with HIV do not seem to have an increased risk for breast, colorectal, or prostate cancer (NCI, 2011). However, because patients frequently see different healthcare providers at a variety of clinical sites, routine screening for non-AIDS-related cancers is often neglected. Since there are no cancer screening guidelines specifically for people living with HIV, it is recommended that healthcare providers screen for cancer in HIV-infected people using the current guidelines for the general population.

Diabetes Mellitus

The incidence of type 2 diabetes mellitus is reported to be as much as 4 times higher among people living with HIV compared to their HIV-negative counterparts. However, it is questionable whether HIV infection is independently associated with diabetes. Current evidence indicates that increased risk for diabetes in persons living with HIV is related more to the use of certain older ARVs, body mass index, and other comorbid conditions such as hepatitis C co-infection, hypertension, and dyslipidemia (Tripathi et al., 2014). Fortunately, research has found that the newer ARVs do not promote glucose intolerance (Rasmusssen et al., 2012).

Current data indicate that hemoglobin A1c may underestimate glycemic control in the HIV population. Therefore, fasting blood sugar or glucose tolerance testing should be used to diagnose and monitor diabetes. People infected with HIV must also have fasting blood sugar testing done before and after the initiation of ARVs (Monroe, Glesby, & Brown, 2015).

Recommendations for preventing diabetes among people aging with HIV are similar to the approach used in uninfected older adults. Healthcare providers should recommend that individuals focus on a lifestyle that includes maintaining a proper body mass index, participating in aerobic exercise and resistance training, and making healthy food choices. Smoking cessation and moderate alcohol intake should also be encouraged (Monroe, Glesby, & Brown, 2015).

Frailty

Frailty is a condition that is related to aging. The most widely used frailty phenotype (FP) was defined by Fried et al. (2001) in a population of older adults (65–101 years), probably HIV negative. The FP requires the presence of three or more of the following five components: unintentional weight loss (10 lb in the past year), self-reported exhaustion, weakness (grip strength), slow walking speed, and low physical activity. Research has found that the presence of frailty can be used to predict health outcomes, including falls, disabilities, loss of independence, and death (Brothers et al., 2014; Piggott et al., 2015).

A higher prevalence of frailty has been observed in people with HIV when compared to their HIV-negative counterparts. The inflammatory effects of HIV infection, HIV-related illness, and the side effects of some antiretroviral drugs have been suggested as possible reasons for the association between frailty and HIV (Piggott et al., 2015). As people live longer with HIV, use of the FP can help healthcare providers measure the impact of illness and treatment on the health status and assess quality of life among people aging with the disease.

Mental Health and Aging with HIV

Neurocognitive Functioning

The American Academy of Neurology recognizes three categories of HIV-associated neurocognitive disorder (HAND): asymptomatic neurocognitive impairment (ANI); mild neurocognitive disorder (MND); and HIV-associated dementia (HAD). ANI is diagnosed when testing shows HIV-associated impairment in cognitive functioning, but daily functioning is not affected. MND, the most common type of HAND, is diagnosed when testing shows HIV-associated impairment in cognitive functioning, and there is mild interference in daily functioning. HAD is diagnosed if testing indicates marked impairment in cognitive functioning. This impairment significantly limits a person's ability to function at work, home, and during social activities (Clifford & Ances, 2013; Sanmarti et al., 2014).

HAND occurs because HIV weakens the immune cells that are protecting the neurons in the brain and causes inflammation that damages these neurons. It is estimated that about 50% of people living with HIV will develop some form of the disease (Hong & Banks, 2015). Risk factors for HAND include age, genetic predisposition, history of injection drug use, CD4 nadir of less than 200 cells, elevated HIV viral load, duration of HIV disease, and existence of comorbidities such as hepatitis C, diabetes, CVD, and depression (McCombe, Vivithanapom, Gill, & Power, 2013). Symptoms of HAND include confusion, forgetfulness, behavioral changes, headaches, gradual weakening and loss of feeling in the arms and legs, problems with cognition or memory, and pain due to nerve damage. These symptoms can range in severity from being very mild to severe and disabling (Clifford & Ances, 2013; Sanmarti et al., 2014).

The single most important treatment for HAND is adherence to ARV therapy that maintains HIV viral suppression (Sanmarti et al., 2014). It is also important that healthcare providers encourage self-care practices to modify factors that contribute to the development of cognitive symptoms in persons aging with HIV. These practices include seeking out treatment for depression, engaging in healthcare maintenance to manage comorbidities (such as hypertension, lipid abnormalities, and diabetes), avoiding non-prescription drugs and excessive alcohol, being socially active, and aerobic exercise. To experience the greatest benefits from exercise, experts recommend at least 30 minutes of activity (such as walking) that raises the heart rate 5 days a week (Fazeli et al., 2014). These self-care practices represent modifiable lifestyle factors that healthcare providers can encourage and tailor to meet the needs of aging HIV-positive adults.

Depression

Depression is a combination of emotional, physical, and behavioral symptoms characterized by sadness, low self-esteem, loss of pleasure, and difficulty functioning. About 7.6% of the general population is considered to be clinically depressed; but rates of depression among older adults living with HIV are as high as 52% (Havlik, 2014; Pratt & Brody, 2014). Moreover, depressed older adults living with HIV have higher levels of suicidal ideation compared to younger adults living with the disease and the general population (Forstein, 2016).

Instruments commonly used for depression screening in HIV primary care clinics are the Patient Health Questionnaire 2 (PHQ-2) and PHQ-9. The PHQ-2 is composed of two questions: Over the past 2 weeks, how often have you been bothered by any of the following problems?

(1) Little interest or pleasure in doing things and (2) Feeling down, depressed, or hopeless. If the PHQ-2 result is negative, further screening is not necessary. If the result is positive, the individual must be screened using the PHQ-9, which has 9 questions. The PHQ-9 takes 2–5 min to complete and is an effective depression screening tool for adults living with HIV (Mitchell, Yadegarfar, Gill, & Stubbs, 2016). To determine if clinical depression is truly evident, further evaluation by a mental health care specialist is required.

Treatment for depression among people living with HIV is consistent with treatment used within the general population, but caution must be used in prescribing antidepressants because of drug–drug interactions. These interactions are more common in older adults living with HIV due to decreased kidney and liver clearance. As always, healthcare providers are advised to take a conservative approach to pharmacology, "start low and go slow" with dosages (Forstein, 2016).

For some people, medication alone may be sufficient to ease their depression; for others, the combination of lifestyle changes, psychotherapy, and/or medication is more effective. Lifestyle changes that improve depression include regular exercise, increased exposure to sunlight, stress management, and improved sleep habits. Psychotherapy, including cognitive behavioral therapy and social support counseling, is often beneficial. When available, community support services can help individuals manage depression by reducing HIV-related stigma, encouraging social engagement, and increasing adherence to care (Forstein, 2016).

Interventions for Successful Aging

Since physical health and mental well-being are primary contributors to successful aging, it is important to identify strategies that improve and sustain functioning as individuals age with HIV. Health promotion is the cornerstone for maintaining health overall, even as persons age with or without a chronic disease. Nakasato and Carnes (2006) summarized this clearly: eat right, eat less, and exercise more. When providing guidance, keep in mind that older persons are not young; therefore, recommendations need to be modified and consideration given to any chronic disease that an individual may be managing. Exercise recommendations need to be tailored to the person's capabilities, and nutrition recommendations congruent with known altered metabolism associated with the presence of a chronic disease. The mental health of the individual cannot be overlooked. Many older individuals experience losses, which can be loss in physical function, loss of loved ones in their social network, and financial concerns. It is important to remember that older persons need to maintain control over their physical and mental health goals no matter what challenges they face (Marquez, Bustamante, Blissmer, & Prohaska, 2009).

Vance, Burrage, Couch, and Raper (2008) proposed hardiness as a strategy to promote successful aging among persons with HIV. Hardiness represents different coping strategies that allow individuals to manage perceived stressful situations or endure difficult situations, and accept life situations with resilience. It is a means of using coping strategies when encountering stressful situations, learning how to react to negative affect, and learning how to model personal behavior after other persons with high hardiness. Some examples are developing well-planned conversations in advance to use during disclosure of HIV status, repeating inspirational phrases to encourage confidence (a form of hardiness), identifying the hardiness behaviors of other persons living with HIV, using positive visualization and positive self-talk, and promoting self-advocacy (self-cheerleader).

Summary

The advent of effective antiretroviral drugs transitioned HIV disease from a death sentence to a chronic illness. Older adults aging with HIV are developing age-related comorbidities that are similar to their HIV-negative counterparts: cardiovascular disease, diabetes, cancer, and osteoporosis. Healthcare providers who work with older HIV-infected adults must not only focus on managing an individual's HIV disease, but also provide patient education about health promotion and prevention activities to reduce the development or progression of other chronic illnesses. Management of HIV among older adults must involve all members of the healthcare team, with the goal focused on improving physical health, mental health, spiritual health, and overall quality of life.

References

Baltes, P. B., & Baltes, M. M. (1990). Psychological perspectives on successful aging: The model of selective optimization with compensation. In P. B. Baltes & M. M. Baltes (Eds.). *Successful aging: Perspectives from the behavioral sciences* (pp. 1–34). United Kingdom: Cambridge University Press. doi:10.1017/CBO9780511665684.003

Brothers, T. D., Kirkland, S., Guaraldi, G., Falutz, J., Theou, O., Johnston, B. L., & Rockwood, K. (2014). Frailty in people aging with human immunodeficiency virus (HIV) infection. *The Journal of Infectious Diseases, 210*(8), 1170–1179. doi:10.1093/infdis/jiu258

Cardoso, S. W., Torres, T. S., Santini-Oliveira, M., Marins, L. M., Veloso, V. G., & Grinsztejn, B. (2013). Aging with HIV: A practical review. *The Brazilian Journal of Infectious Diseases, 17*(4), 464–479. doi:10.1016/j.bjid.2012.11.007

Centers for Disease Control and Prevention [CDC]. (2016). *HIV among people aged 50 and over.* Retrieved from http://www.cdc.gov/hiv/pdf/group/age/olderamericans/cdc-hiv-older-americans.pdf

Clifford, D. B., & Ances, B. M. (2013). HIV-associated neurocognitive disorder (HAND). *Lancet Infectious Diseases, 13*(11), 976–986. doi:10.1016/S1473-3099(13)70269-X

Costa, L. A., & Almeida, A. G. (2015). Cardiovascular disease associated with immunodeficiency virus: A review. *Portuguese Journal of Cardiology, 34*(7–8), 479–491. doi:10.1016/j.repc.2015.03.005

Department of Health and Human Services. (2016). *Guidelines for the prevention and treatment of opportunistic infections in HIV-infected adults and adolescents: Human papillomavirus disease.* Retrieved from https://aidsinfo.nih.gov/guidelines/html/4/adult-and-adolescent-oi-prevention-and-treatment-guidelines/343/hpv

Donnellan, C., & O'Neill, D. (2014). Baltes' SOC model of successful ageing as a potential framework for stroke rehabilitation. *Disability and Rehabilitation, 36*(5), 424–429. doi:10.3109/09638288.2013.793412

Fazeli, P. L., Woods, S. P., Heaton, R. K., Umlauf, A., Gouauz, B., Rosario, D. … HNRP Group. (2014). An active lifestyle is associated with better neurocognitive functioning in adults living with HIV infection. *Journal of Neurovirology, 20*, 233–242. doi:10.1007/s13365-014-0240-z

Forstein, M. (2016). *Depression in the aging HIV infected population.* Retrieved from http://hiv-age.org/2016/01/26/depression-in-the-aging-hiv-infected-population/

Fried, L. P., Tangen, C. M., Walston, J., Newman, A. B., Hirsch, C. Gottdiener, J. ... McBurnie, M. A. (2001). Frailty in older adults: Evidence for a phenotype. *The Journals of Gerontology. Series A, Biological Sciences and Medical Sciences, 56*(3), M146–M156. doi:10.1093/gerona/56.3.M146

Grulich, A. E., van Leeuwen, M. T., Falster, M. O., & Vajdic, C. M. (2007). Incidence of cancers in people with HIV/AIDS compared with immunosuppressed transplant recipients: A meta-analysis. *Lancet, 370,* 59–67. Retrieved from http://www.natap.org/2007/HIV/PIIS0140673607610502.pdf

Havlik, R. J. (2014). Multimorbidity and depression in HIV-infected older adults. *Psychology and AIDS Exchange Newsletter.* Retrieved from http://www.apa.org/pi/aids/resources/exchange/2014/01/multi-morbidity.aspx

Hong, S., & Banks, W. A. (2015). Role of the immune system in HIV-associated neuroinflammation and neurocognitive implications. *Brain, Behavior, and Immunity, 45,* 1–12. doi:10.1016/j.bbi.2014.10.008

Kahana, E., & Kahana, B. (1996). Conceptual and empirical advances in understanding aging well through proactive adaptation. In V. Bengtson (Ed.), *Adulthood, and aging: Research on continuities and discontinuities* (pp. 18–40). New York, NY: Springer.

Kahana, E., & Kahana, B. (2001). Successful aging among people with HIV/AIDS. *Journal of Clinical Epidemiology, 54,* S53–S56. doi:10.1016/S0895-4356(01)00447-4

Mallon, P. W. (2014). Aging with HIV: Osteoporosis and fractures. *Current Opinion in HIV/AIDS, 9*(4). doi:10.1097/COH.0000000000000080

Manner, I. W., Baekken, M., Oektedalen, O., & Os, I. (2012). Hypertension and antihypertensive treatment in HIV-infected individuals. A longitudinal cohort study. *Blood Pressure, 21,* 11–319. doi:10.3109/08037051.2012.680742

Marquez, D. X., Bustamante, E. E., Blissmer, B. J., & Prohaska, T. R. (2009). Health promotion for successful aging. *American Journal of Life Style Medicine, 3*(1), 12–19. doi:10.1177/1559827608325200

Martin, P., Kelly, N., Kahana, B., Kahana, E., Wilcox, B. J., Wilcox, D. C., & Poon, L. W. (2015). Defining successful aging: A tangible or elusive concept. *The Gerontologist, 55*(1), 14–25. doi:10.1093/geront/gnu044

McCombe, J. A., Vivithanaporn, P., Gill, J. J., & Power, C. (2013). Predictors of symptomatic HIV-associated neurocognitive disorders in universal health care. *HIV Medicine, 14*(2), 99–107. doi:10.1111/j.1468-1293.2012.01043.x

Mitchell, A. J., Yadegarfar, M., Gill, J., & Stubbs, B. (2016). Case finding and screening clinical utility of the Patient Health Questionnaire (PHQ-9 and PHQ-2) for depression in primary care: A diagnostic meta-analysis of 40 studies. *British Journal of Psychiatry Open, 2*(2) 127–138. doi:10.1192/bjpo.bp.115.001685

Monroe, A. K., Fu, W., Zikusoka, M. N., Jacobson, L. P., Witt, M. D., Palella, F. J. ... Brown, T. T. (2015). Low-density lipoprotein cholesterol levels and statin treatment by HIV status among multicenter AIDS cohort study men. *AIDS Research and Human Retroviruses 31*(6), 593–602. doi:10.1089/aid.2014.0126

Monroe, A. K., Glesby, M. J., & Brown, T. W. (2015). Diagnosing and managing diabetes in HIV-infected patients: Current concepts. *Clinical Infectious Disease, 60,* 453–462. doi:10.1093/cid/ciu779

Nakasato, Y. R., & Carners, B. A. (2006). Health promotion in older adults. Promoting successful aging in primary care settings. *Geriatrics, 61*(4), 27–31.

National Cancer Institute [NCI]. (2011). *HIV infection and cancer risk.* Retrieved from http://www.cancer.gov/about-cancer/causes-prevention/risk/infectious-agents/hiv-fact-sheet

National Cancer Institute [NCI]. (2015). *HPV and cancer.* Retrieved from http://www.cancer.gov/about-cancer/causes-prevention/risk/infectious-agents/hpv-fact-sheet

Nery, M. W., Martelli, C. M., Silveira, E. A., de Sousa, C. A., de Oliveira Falco, M., de Castro, A. C. ... Turchi, M. D. (2013). Cardiovascular risk assessment: A comparison of the Framingham, PROCAM, and DAD equation in HIV-infected persons. *The Scientific World Journal, 3,* 9. doi:10.1155/2013/969281

Palacios, R., Pascual, J., Cabrera, E., Lebrón, J. M., Guerrero-León, M.A., del Arco, A. … Santos, J. (2014). Lung cancer in HIV-infected patients. *International Journal of STD & AIDS, 25*(14), 239–243. doi:10.1177/0956462413499317

Piggott, D. A., Varadhan, R., Mehta, S. H. Brown, T. T., Li, H., Walston, J. D. … Kirk, G. D. (2015). Frailty, inflammation, and mortality among persons aging with HIV infection and injection drug use. *Journal of Gerontology, 70*(12), 1542–1547. doi:10.1093/gerona/glv107

Pratt, L. A., & Brody, D. J. (2014). *Depression in the U.S. household population, 2009–2012.* National Center for Health Statistics. Brief no. 172. Retrieved from http://www.cdc.gov/nchs/data/databriefs/db172.pdf

Rasmussen, L. D., Mathiesen, E. R., Kronborg, G., Pedersen, C., Gerstoft, J., & Obel, N. (2012). Risk of diabetes mellitus in persons with and without HIV: A Danish nationwide population-based cohort study. *PLOS One, 7*(9). doi:10.1371/journal.pone.0044575

Rowe, J. W., & Kahn, R. L. (1998). *Successful aging.* New York, NY: Oxford University Press.

Rueda, S., Law, S., & Rourke, S. B. (2014). Psychosocial, mental health, and behavioral issues of aging with HIV. *Current Opinion in HIV/AIDS, 9*(4), 325–331. doi:10.1097/COH.0000000000000071

Sadlier, C., Rowley, D., Morley, D., Surah, S., O'Dea, S., Delamere, S. … Bergin, C. (2014). Prevalence of human papillomavirus in men who have sex with men in the era of an effective vaccine: A call to act. *HIV Medicine, 15*(8), 499–504. doi:10.1111/hiv.12150

Samji, H., Cescon, A., Hogg, R. S., Modur, S. P., Althoff, K. N., Buchacz, K. … Gange, S. J. (2013). Closing the gap: Increases in life expectancy among treated HIV-positive individuals in the United States and Canada. *PLOS One, 13*(8), 1–8. Retrieved from http://journals.plos.org/plosone/article/asset?id=10.1371%2Fjournal.pone.0081355.PDF

Sanmarti, M., Ibáñez, L., Huertas, S., Badenes, D., Dalmau, D., Slevein, M. … Jaen, A. (2014). HIV associated neurocognitive disorders. *Journal of Molecular Psychiatry, 2*(2), 10. doi:10.1186/2049-9256-2-2

Short, C. S., Shaw, S. G., Fisher, M. J., Walker-Bone, K., & Gilleece, U. C. (2014). Prevalence of and risk factors for osteoporosis and fracture among a male HIV-infected population in the UK. *International Journal of STD & AIDS, 25*(2), 113–121. doi:10.1177/0956462413492714std.sagepub.com

Silverberg, M. J., Lau, B., Achenbach, C. J., Jing, Y., Althoff, K. N., D'Souoza, G. … Dubrow, R. (2015). Cumulative incidence of cancer among persons with HIV in North America: A cohort study. *Annals of Internal Medicine, 163*(7), 507–518. doi:10.7326/M14-2768

Topaz, M., Troutman-Jordan, M., & MacKenzie, M. (2014). Construction, deconstruction, and reconstruction: The roots of successful aging theories. *Nursing Science Quarterly, 27*(3), 226–233. doi:10.1177/0894318414534484

Triant, V. A. (2013). Cardiovascular disease and HIV infection. *Current HIV/AIDS Report, 10*(3), 199–206. doi:10.1007/s11904-013-0168-6

Tripathi, A., Liese, A. D., Jerrell, J. M., Zhange, J., Rizvi, A. A., Albrecht, H., & Duffus, W. A. (2014). Incidence of diabetes mellitus in a population based cohort of HIV-infected and non-infected persons: The impact of clinical and therapeutic factors over time. *Diabetic Medicine, 10*, 1185–1193. doi:10.1111/dme.1245

Vance, D. E., Burrage, J., Couch, A., & Raper, J. (2008). Promoting successful aging with HIV through hardiness: Implications for nursing practice and research. *Journal of Gerontological Nursing, 34*(6), 22–29. Retrieved from http://www.healio.com/nursing/journals/jgn

Index

Note: Page numbers followed by *f* and *t* indicate figures and tables respectively.

© Springer International Publishing AG 2017
F.M. Parks et al. (eds.), *HIV/AIDS in Rural Communities*,
DOI 10.1007/978-3-319-56239-1